The Vulva Owner's Manual on Birth Control

The Vulva Owner's Manual on Birth Control

Finding *Your* Best Option for Contraception

Kristine Shields MSN, DrPH

ISBN 978-1-7353742-1-5

Publisher's Cataloging-in-Publication Data

Names: Shields, Kristine, author.
Title: The vulva owner's guide to birth control : finding your best option for contraception / Kristine Shields MSN, DrPH.
Series: The Vulva Owner's Manuals
Description: Includes bibliographical references. | Philadelphia, PA: Blackfox Communications, 2020.
Identifiers: LCCN: 2020913898| ISBN: 978-1-7353742-1-5 (pbk.) | 978-1-735374-0-8 (ebook)
Subjects: LCSH Contraceptives--Popular works. | Contraceptive drugs. | Birth control. | Fertility. | BISAC HEALTH & FITNESS / Women's Health | SELF-HELP / Gender & Sexuality | YOUNG ADULT NONFICTION / Health & Daily Living / Sexuality & Pregnancy
Classification: LCC RG137 .S55 2020 | DDC 613.9/43--dc23

The Vulva Owner's Manuals

The Vulva Owner's Manuals are written to assist women and men find concise, helpful information about the reproductive health issues occurring in their lives. The books contain knowledge that is usually available online or in the medical literature. But because so much information is available in so many places, online searches can be time-consuming and result in conflicting advice. The Vulva Owner's Manuals seek to clarify and consolidate the medical information women and men need to make healthy decisions about their bodies.

Kristine Shields, the author of the guidebooks, is a Doctor of Public Health and a Women's Health Nurse Practitioner. Her career is dedicated to women's health and empowerment. From her education, clinical practice, and reviews of current research, she compiles the most accurate, positive, and helpful information in one place — to inform, comfort, and empower you to be safe, sane, and healthy.

Knowledge and practice in health care are constantly changing as new research and experience impact our understanding. Recommendations for care evolve. We all seek to protect and enhance our own and our loved one's health and safety. When confused or uncertain, seek advice from trusted sources and health care professionals. The information in this book is not intended to substitute for or replace advice from a licensed medical professional. The author disclaims any liability arising directly or indirectly from the use of this book.

Note to the Reader: Because the subject of the manual is avoiding pregnancy, throughout this book the word 'intercourse' will mean penis-in-vagina intercourse unless otherwise noted. The author recognizes that there are many other types of intercourse.

Contents

The Vulva Owner's Manual	i
Birth Control in Perspective	1
Meet the Millers	7
How to Choose a Birth Control Method	10
Decision Tree #1: Marion and Dave	16
Tubal Ligation	17
Vasectomy	19
Decision Tree #2: Liz and Josh	23
Breastfeeding for Birth Control	24
Spermicide	28
Diaphragm or Cervical Cap	30
Cervical Sponge	32
Male Condom	34
Internal (Female) Condom	37
Decision Tree #3: Daphne	42
Oral Contraceptives ("the Pill")	49
Vaginal Ring	50

Skin Patch 51
Progestin-only Pills (Mini-pills) 54
Birth Control Injection (the Shot) 55
Hormonal Rod Implants 57
No Birth Control Method 62
Withdrawal 63
Fertility Awareness or Natural Family Planning 65
Copper IUD 68
Hormonal IUDs 71
Emergency Contraception (EC) 80
The Cost of Birth Control 87
Choosing Your Birth Control Method 89

Resources 93
Appendix I: Birth Control Method Chart 96
Appendix II: Birth Control Method Worksheet 116
Appendix III: Birth Control Method Quiz 129
References 135
Author's Note 138
Author Biography 140

Birth Control in Perspective

As a Women's Health Nurse Practitioner, I've been helping women choose their method of birth control since 1982. Plus, I've used a number of them myself. It has been my pleasure to help women find the method that meets their needs wherever they are in their life's journey. As lives change, birth control methods (BCMs) can change too. Planning when, and when not, to have a baby is an important part of being a responsible, healthy, sexually active woman. The methods of birth control we'll discuss in this book can help you prevent an unplanned pregnancy, have a healthy sex life, and have a baby when you want one. I'll give you the questions you should ask yourself so you can determine which BCM is right for you, and we'll look at all the methods in detail.

A Short History of Birth Control

We are fortunate to have a variety of BCMs to choose from today. A quick review of the history of contraception will remind us of how lucky we are.

Birth control, also called contraception, family planning, and fertility control, allows men and women to decide if and when they want to have children.

Birth control methods work by:

- preventing ovulation (the release of an egg by the ovary),
- preventing sperm from reaching the egg,
- preventing sperm from being able to fertilize an egg,
- preventing a uterine environment that could nurture a fertilized egg.

People have been trying to have control over whether and when they choose to have babies for as long as recorded history.

- The use of condoms can be traced all the way back to 11,000 BCE as seen in cave paintings in France.
- Pastes combining dates, honey, sour milk, acacia gum, and herbs were put into the vagina — some of which actually worked!
- The giant fennel herb, called silphium, was found to help prevent pregnancy. It was so popular that it became extinct!
- The first condoms made from rubber appeared in the U.S. in the 1800s — that's why they are sometimes called "rubbers."

- Condoms first became legal in the U.S. in 1918 — and during the 1920s the birth rate decreased by half!

In addition to preventing pregnancy, condoms were used to prevent sexually transmitted infections, especially syphilis, for which no effective cure was known until the 1940s.

Effective BCMs allow women and men to plan when they will have children and to prepare emotionally, socially, and financially for the care of those children. Family planning also contributes to improved health outcomes for babies, children, women, and families.[1]

Who Needs Birth Control?

Most people agree that family planning is one of the 10 great public health achievements of the 20th century.[2] Yet, of all the pregnancies that occurred around the world between 2010 and 2014, about 44% were unintended.[3]

Birth control methods: [4,5,6]

- **help women** avoid unplanned pregnancies. Worldwide, over 400 million unplanned pregnancies have been averted since family planning programs began their work in the 1900s. By preventing high-risk pregnancies and unsafe abortions, many women's lives have been saved.

- **help men** avoid unplanned pregnancies. Fathers and mothers are equally responsible for providing physical, emotional, and financial support for their children.
- **help children** survive. If all children were born at least 2 years apart, 3 to 4 million childhood deaths would be avoided worldwide.
- **help relationships** evolve. Intimacy and sexual pleasure develop in an atmosphere devoid of worries about an unplanned pregnancy.
- **help families** thrive. Families who can determine the number and spacing of their children are better able to provide quality food, clothing, housing, education, and emotional support.
- **help countries** prosper. Those that provide access and education about family planning have improved economic and health outcomes.
- **help the earth** survive. If couples have fewer children in the future, the world's current population of almost 8 billion people will avert doubling in less than 50 years and demands on resources such as food, water, fossil fuels, and fertile soil will be less.

Both external (male) condoms and internal (female) condoms continue to be one of the most widely used contraceptives and one of the few methods that provide protection from sexually transmitted infections (STIs).

A wide variety of effective birth control methods are now available.

Women and men use birth control methods to:

- prevent pregnancy,
- plan the interval of time between pregnancies,
- prevent the spread of sexually transmitted infections,
- regulate menstrual cycles,
- decrease the risk, occurrence, and effect of certain conditions and diseases.

A woman's need for birth control changes throughout the course of her lifetime.

- Teenagers or young adults who are considering becoming sexually active should prepare themselves with information about the menstrual cycle and how it relates to fertility. They should understand the types of BCMs that are available and the advantages and disadvantages of each.
- Women in their childbearing years should think about when and if they want to have children. Becoming a parent should be a choice, not an expectation — and not a surprise! Knowing if and when they might want to conceive a child can help them decide what BCM they should use.

- Women who are postpartum or breastfeeding have different needs than women who are close to menopause but still fertile.
- Women with certain medical conditions may be limited in the types of BCMs they can safely use. Discussing your medical history and contraceptive needs with your health care provider can help you choose the method that is best for you.

All individuals should reassess their risk of contracting STIs as their relationships change, seeking open and honest conversation with their partner(s) about their needs. People who are sexually active with more than one partner or whose partner is not monogamous should be tested for STIs annually or anytime they develop any symptoms (vaginal discharge, itching, pain).

Meet the Millers

We'll use the women in the Miller family as examples of how our needs and wants change over the course of our lifetimes.

- **Marion** is pregnant and soon to deliver. She and her husband have decided they do not want any more children after this one, their third, is born.

- **Liz** is Marion's younger sister. She has one infant and would like to have more.

- **Daphne** is Marion and Liz's aunt. She is 49 years old and does not plan to have any more children. She is not currently sexually active.

- **Jade** is Daphne's daughter. She is 18 and wants birth control advice from her mom.

- **Daniella**, while not really a Miller, is Jade's best friend. She moved in with Daphne and Jade when her birth family struggled to accept her as a woman. She is considered one of the family.

Each of these women is struggling to find the BCM that is right for her. Choosing the right method can be difficult and each option has advantages and disadvantages. You may be surprised by the Miller family's decisions!

The Challenge of Choosing

Now let's listen in on the Millers discussing their birth control plans:

It's after the baby shower, and the family is scooping up wrapping paper and emptying the punch bowl. Marion, who is due to deliver her third baby in the next three weeks, collapses into a chair. "Whew!" she says. "I'm ready for this baby to come out! I don't want to be pregnant anymore — but I'm a little sad that this will be my last one. Such a special time."

Daphne, Marion's aunt, responds, "I didn't know you made that decision, Marion."

"Yup," says Marion, "this is it. Dave's getting a vasectomy after we're sure this baby's healthy."

"How about you, Liz? You planning to have any more kids?" asks Daphne to Marion's younger sister.

Liz smiles shyly. "Oh yes, I want at least one more. I'd like Nora to have a little brother or sister. Josh agrees — he's not ready to get snipped, anyway. If he'll ever be ... Right now, I'm breastfeeding, but I know I have to choose a birth control method soon."

"See, Mom," says Daphne's daughter, Jade. "People can talk about birth control without getting all freaky!"

Now Daphne is blushing and everyone's giggling. Daniella is shaking her head. "Guess I'll have to figure that out, too."

Obviously, these five women have different needs when it comes to controlling their fertility. Who will choose what method? And how will they decide? Let's find out.

How to Choose a Birth Control Method

Recommendation #1: Consider your priorities.

There are many factors to consider, which I've listed in Table 1. Think about all of them before deciding. No method of birth control is perfect. Ask yourself the following questions when trying to decide which method would work best for you. Which issues are most important to you?

TABLE 1. QUESTIONS TO CONSIDER WHEN CHOOSING A BIRTH CONTROL METHOD	
Do I want kids someday?	Should I choose a permanent or a temporary method? Am I sure about my decision to have or not have children?
Impact of a pregnancy	How would an unplanned pregnancy affect my life? Could I handle having a baby or an abortion?

TABLE 1. QUESTIONS TO CONSIDER WHEN CHOOSING A BIRTH CONTROL METHOD	
Efficacy	How effective is this method in preventing pregnancy?
Convenience	How easy is this method to use?
Cost	What can I afford? Do I have insurance that pays for contraception?
Control	Do I want to rely on my partner to use the BCM or do I want to be in control?
Accessibility	Can I buy it at the pharmacy or do I need to see a health care provider?
Side effects	What kinds of unwanted side effects might occur? What can I put up with in order to prevent pregnancy? Could there be side effects I would like?
STI protection	What is my risk for getting a sexually transmitted infection
Reversibility	If I use it now, can I get pregnant later? How soon will I be able to get pregnant after I stop using this method?

TABLE 1. QUESTIONS TO CONSIDER WHEN CHOOSING A BIRTH CONTROL METHOD	
Effect on my periods	Will it make my period heavier/lighter or more regular or irregular? Might this method cause my periods to stop? Is that good or bad?
Non-contraceptive benefits	Are there physical advantages to some methods, like an effect on my period, acne, menstrual cramps, or my risk of getting cancer in the future?
Contraindications	Do I have medical conditions that might affect my choice, like breastfeeding, obesity, allergies to latex, or blood disorders?
Preferences	Some people don't like to use hormones. Some people prefer methods that prevent conception rather than prevent implantation. Some don't want to remember to take a pill every day. Others don't like getting shots. What other preferences might you and your partner(s) need to talk about?

Recommendation #2: Choose the most effective method of birth control that you are likely to use successfully.

Stopping a method of contraception because you or your partner don't like to use it or because of side effects causes a significant number of unintended pregnancies each year. There are many methods to choose from. Really think about which one fits your personality and your lifestyle the most.

Generally speaking, the methods that need the smallest amount of attention are the ones that people use successfully the longest.

For example, Table 2 lists some of the popular BCMs that are widely used. (See Appendix I for a list of all the BCMs available to you.) The number represents the percentage of women (and men) who started to use this method and continued to use it for at least one year.

TABLE 2. CONTINUATION OF BIRTH CONTROL METHODS DURING A ONE-YEAR PERIOD

Birth control method	Percent of couples who still used this method after one year
Hormonal rod implant	84%
Hormonal IUD	80%
Copper IUD	78%

TABLE 2. CONTINUATION OF BIRTH CONTROL METHODS DURING A ONE-YEAR PERIOD	
Birth control method	**Percent of couples who still used this method after one year**
Hormonal pills, patch, or vaginal ring	67%
Diaphragm	57%
Birth control injection or shot	56%
Fertility awareness	47%
Male condom	43%
Internal condom	41%

As you can see, the methods that couples used for the longest period of time required the least amount of their attention. Keep that in mind when choosing your method. Also be aware that a BCM used perfectly (consistently and correctly) is more effective than the same method used incorrectly or inconsistently. Again, the methods that need the smallest amount of attention are also the most effective.

The Millers Make Their Decisions

Let's see how each of the Miller women is making her decision.

Marion and Dave

Marion is due to have her third baby in a few weeks. She and her husband, Dave, have decided they do not want any more children in the future. They are very sure about this decision.

Marion and Dave's priorities:

- High efficacy — should I choose a permanent or a long-acting temporary method?
- Cost — what can I afford? What does my insurance plan cover?

[See Decision Tree #1]

Decision Tree #1: Marion and Dave

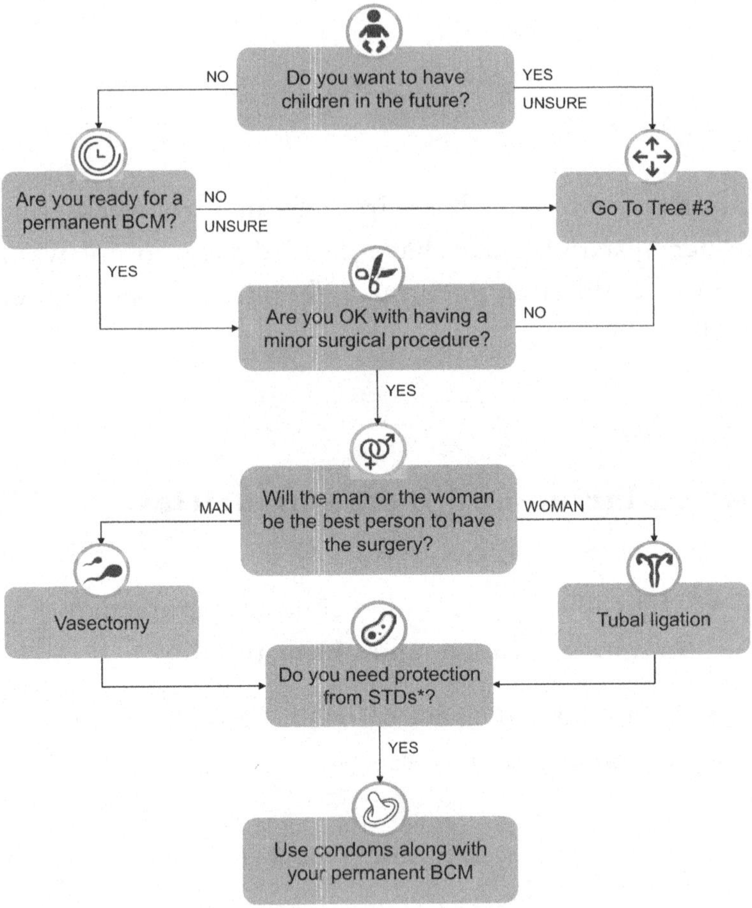

*You don't need protection from sexually transmitted diseases (STDs) if you and your partner(s) have tested STD-free and are only having sex with each other.

Marion and Dave's options:

Tubal Ligation

A tubal ligation is a surgical procedure during which a doctor will close off the woman's fallopian tubes (the passageways that allow the egg released from the ovary to travel to the uterus). You will still ovulate (release an egg every month), but the egg won't get to the uterus (it will be absorbed by the body) and so it will not be in a position to get fertilized by sperm.

The surgery is usually done through a small incision or two in your abdomen through which instruments are passed to tie off or clamp the tubes. You will be given anesthesia so you won't feel the operation and you will usually go home the same day. The procedure results in permanent closure of the fallopian tubes. Attempts to reopen the tubes are not very successful, so you must be sure you are finished with having children before deciding to have a tubal ligation.

Pros:

- Almost 100% effective, lasts forever, usually paid for by insurance, no need to worry about an unexpected pregnancy.

Cons:

- Can't usually be reversed if you change your mind about wanting more children, expensive one-time cost if not covered by insurance, doesn't protect against STIs.

Side effects:

- Short-term bleeding or cramping after the procedure. Usually no long-term side effects.

Vasectomy

A vasectomy is a surgical procedure during which a doctor will close off the man's vas deferens (the tubes that carry sperm from the testicles to the penis) so that the fluid he ejaculates does not contain sperm. This procedure takes about 30 minutes and is usually performed in a doctor's office or clinic with local anesthesia (numbing of the testicles). You must use an additional method of birth control for the first two months after the procedure to allow time for the sperm that are already in the ejaculate fluid to be gone. Then the fluid is tested to be sure the vasectomy was effective and there are no more sperm getting through. Having a vasectomy does not change your sex drive or ability to have an erection or ejaculation.

Pros:

- Almost 100% effective, lasts forever, usually paid for by insurance, no need to worry about an unexpected pregnancy. A vasectomy is both cheaper and safer for a man than a tubal ligation is for a woman.

Cons:

- Requires surgery, can't usually be reversed if you change your mind about wanting more children, expensive one-time cost if not covered by insurance, doesn't protect against STIs.

Side effects:

- Short-term bleeding, bruising, tenderness in the scrotum. Usually no long-term side effects.

• • •

Marion and Dave's decision: Vasectomy

Because it is safer for Dave to have a vasectomy than it is for Marion to have a tubal ligation, together they decide that Dave will schedule an appointment with his doctor to have a vasectomy soon after the new baby is born.

Liz and Josh

Liz had a baby three months ago and continues to breastfeed her baby exclusively (no formula supplements). She and her husband are planning to have more children in the future. Right now, she is relying on breastfeeding to prevent ovulation. (Exclusive breastfeeding can prevent the release of an egg from the ovary for up to 6 months.) But Liz knows she has to start using a birth control method soon in order to make sure she doesn't get pregnant again until she is ready.

Liz knows that taking estrogen is not recommended for use while breastfeeding because it could decrease her milk supply. She knows that progestin-only birth control methods are very effective. Even though progestin is considered safe to take while breastfeeding, Liz wants to stay away from medications, supplements, or alcohol that could get to her baby through her breast milk.

Liz and Josh's priorities:

- Reversibility and time to return of fertility — if I use it now, can I get pregnant later? How soon will I be able to get pregnant after I stop using the method?
- Contraindications — do I have medical conditions that might affect my choice, like breastfeeding, obesity, allergies to latex, or blood disorders?
- Preferences — am I okay with using hormonal methods?
- Impact — how would an unplanned pregnancy affect my life? Could I handle having a baby or an abortion?

[See Decision Tree #2]

Decision Tree #2: Liz and Josh

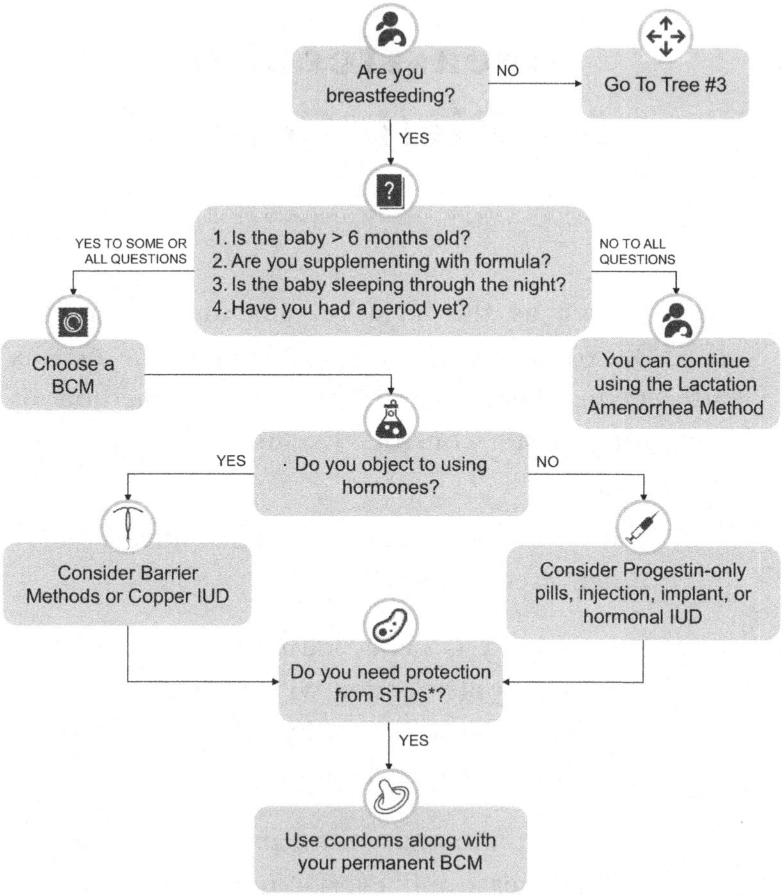

*You don't need protection from sexually transmitted diseases (STDs) if you and your partner(s) have tested STD-free and are only having sex with each other.

Liz and Josh's options:

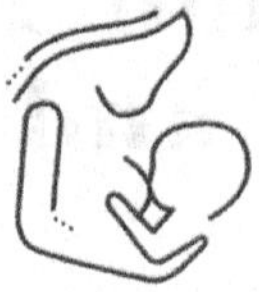

Breastfeeding for Birth Control

Also known as the lactation amenorrhea method (LAM), exclusive breastfeeding for up to six months after giving birth can be an effective method of temporary birth control. Exclusive breastfeeding means that:

- it's been less than 6 months since you delivered your baby,
- your baby is being fed only breast milk — no supplementing with formula — or at least the vast majority (about 85%) of feedings are breastfeeds,
- you are nursing your baby or pumping your breast milk every 4 to 6 hours, even throughout the night,
- and your period has not yet started.

If the above are all true for you, you have a less than 2% risk of getting pregnant (only 2 out of 100 women would get pregnant under these circumstances).[7] That means LAM is about as good as using a condom correctly and consistently to prevent pregnancy.

Under these conditions, your nursing hormones suppress the release of eggs from the ovary. But once the baby is six months old, the chances of ovulating become too high and you must use another method of birth control to prevent pregnancy. If you get your period before six months, you will know you have begun to ovulate and should use another birth control method.

Pros:

- Safe and effective
- No cost
- Does not interfere with breastfeeding

Cons:

- Only effective until fertility returns
- No protection from STIs

Side effects:

- None

Barrier methods

Barrier methods are not as highly effective as some other birth control methods like hormone-containing methods or IUDs. But barrier methods generally have fewer side effects and a low one-time cost, and some can be obtained without a prescription.

Pros:

- They are safe, simple, and convenient.
- They can be inserted ahead of time so it is not too disruptive to sexual activity.
- Some (male and internal condoms, spermicides, and sponges) do not require a visit to your health care provider to get a prescription.
- Some (male and internal condoms) protect against sexually transmitted infections (STIs).

Cons:

- They must be used every time you have sex.
- Some methods (diaphragm, cervical cap) require a visit to your health care provider to get a prescription.
- They are less effective at preventing pregnancy than some other birth control methods.

Side effects:

- In some people, certain barrier methods or spermicides may cause irritation of the vagina or penis.

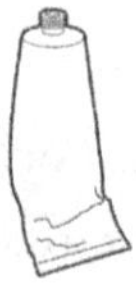

Spermicide

Spermicides are creams, gels, foams, or films that contain chemical agents that interfere with a sperm's ability to fertilize an egg. They can be acquired at pharmacies or stores that sell personal products like condoms and tampons. No prescription is required to buy spermicide and many brands are available. Most products contain nonoxynol-9 or a similar ingredient that kills or disables sperm. Packaging usually includes an applicator with which a woman inserts the product into her vagina within one hour or less of having sexual intercourse. If used by itself for contraception, about 28 out of 100 women will get pregnant. That rate is not good enough to recommend the use of spermicides alone for contraception. However, when used with other barrier methods, spermicides increase their effectiveness. It is recommended to use spermicide and condoms together to reduce the risk of pregnancy and STIs; diaphragms and cervical caps require the use of spermicide to be effective. Spermicides do not protect against STIs.

In May 2020, the FDA approved a new non-hormonal, spermicidal birth control gel called Phexxi. Testing indicated that about 14 out of every 100 women could get pregnant using this product alone, which is better than the spermicides already on the market but still not as effective as other BCMs. Rather than killing the sperm with chemical agents, Phexxi works by counteracting the sperm's alkaline effect on the vaginal ph. Sperm become inactivated as the vagina retains its acidic nature. It's a nifty way to prevent pregnancy and maintain a healthy vaginal ph at the same time. But there has been no reported protection from STIs, so condoms would still be needed outside of a secure monogamous sexual relationship. Phexxi requires a prescription, is more expensive than other spermicides, and is not recommended for women who experience recurrent urinary tract infections.

Spermicides retain the pros, cons, and side effects of barrier methods unless otherwise noted in this section.

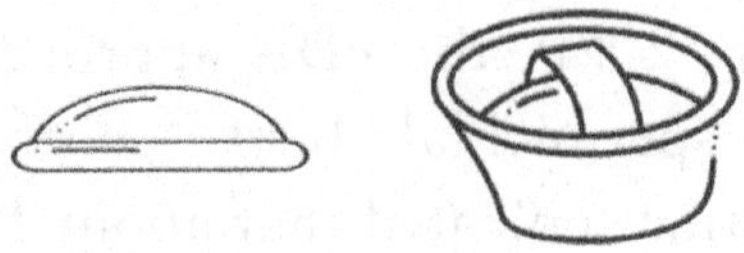

Diaphragm or Cervical Cap

The diaphragm and the cervical cap are similar. They both require a visit to your health care provider or clinic so they can be fitted for you correctly. They both must be inserted into your vagina to cover your cervix before every act of intercourse. They both provide a barrier to prevent sperm from getting into the uterus through the cervix. Any sperm that might get past them is killed by the spermicide. The diaphragm and the cervical cap must be used with spermicide to be effective.

The diaphragm is a thin flexible rubber cup that fits into the back of your vagina, covering your cervix. You put spermicide in and around the rim before you insert it. If used correctly every time, the risk of getting pregnant is low (about 6 out of every 100 women would get pregnant in a year). But because it is not always used correctly, the pregnancy rate among all diaphragm users is about 16 out of 100 women. A new one-size-fits-most diaphragm is now on the market. Ask your health care provider if it might be appropriate for you.

The cervical cap is a smaller, bowl-shaped silicone cup that fits snugly against your cervix. You put spermicide in and around the rim before you insert it. Among all cervical cap users, about 14 out of 100 women who have never given birth will become pregnant each year. If they've had a baby before, about 29 out of 100 women will become pregnant each year.

Diaphragms and caps come in different sizes to accurately fit different women. Your health care provider can make sure that the one you choose fits you correctly. They'll teach you how to insert and remove it correctly too. Neither you nor your partner will feel it inside you when it is in place. The diaphragm and cap can be inserted before intercourse (the diaphragm can be inserted up to 6 hours before sex and the cap can be inserted up to 24 hours before sex), but each should not be removed until at least six hours after the last act of intercourse. The diaphragm costs about $15 to $75 and the cap costs $60 to $80, depending on the cost of the visit. With care (washing and drying and storing it correctly), your diaphragm or cap can last about two years. You should be refitted if you gain or lose more than ten pounds or after a pregnancy and delivery.

See the pros, cons, and side effects listed in the section on barrier methods.

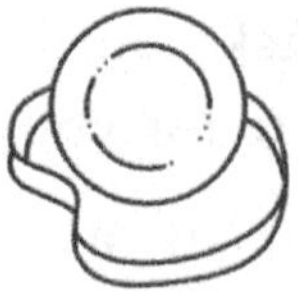

Cervical Sponge

The cervical sponge can be bought at the pharmacy, supermarket, or clinic without a prescription. The soft sponge is made of foam that contains spermicide. A package of three sponges costs about $9 to $15.

You insert the sponge into your vagina to cover your cervix before you have intercourse. You can insert it up to 24 hours before sex, and it must stay in place for six hours afterward. Then you remove it by pulling on the attached loop. It cannot be felt by you or your partner during sex. The sponge provides a barrier to prevent sperm from getting to the cervix, and the spermicide kills sperm. Each sponge is disposable — one sponge can only be used one time.

The sponge is not as effective as some other methods of birth control. It is more effective if you have never had a pregnancy and delivery. If used correctly every time, about 6 out of every 100 women will get pregnant in a year (20 out of 100 women if they've had a baby before). But because it is not always used correctly the pregnancy rate among all sponge users is about 16 out of 100 women (32 out of 100 women if they've previously given birth).

See the pros, cons, and side effects in the section on barrier methods.

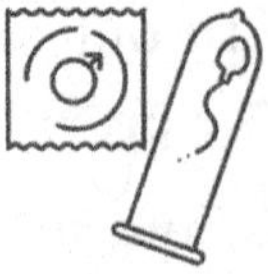

Male Condom

Condoms are thin covers made of latex, silicone, or polyurethane that are put on over the erect penis with every act of intercourse. The condom acts as a barrier that prevents sperm from getting into the vagina. Condoms protect against pregnancy and most sexually transmitted infections (STIs).

(Natural condoms are made from animal intestines and have larger microscopic pores than other condoms. The pores are small enough to stop sperm but not small enough to stop viruses. Therefore, natural condoms protect against pregnancy but not against STIs.)

Condoms that are packaged with spermicide are not recommended because they may be irritating. However, you can use spermicide that you buy separately to improve your protection against pregnancy.

Like all barrier methods, condoms work better to prevent pregnancy when you use them correctly every time. If condoms are always used correctly, only 2 out of 100 women will get pregnant each year. If condoms are not always used correctly, 15 out of 100 women will get pregnant each year. If the condom comes off during intercourse, you should consider taking emergency contraception (EC) as soon as possible within five days (see the section on EC).

Pros:

- Condoms are safe, simple, easily accessible, and low cost (or free from some clinics).
- Condoms have few side effects.
- Anyone can buy condoms in a store without a prescription.
- People who use condoms feel their experiences are just as pleasurable as people who don't.[8]
- Condoms protect against STIs. Remember, you are four times more likely to get an STI than you are to get pregnant.

Cons:

- You must use a condom each time you have sex.
- Condoms are not as effective at preventing pregnancy as some other birth control methods.

- Using condoms requires cooperation from the male partner.
- Both partners should be in agreement about using this method.

Side effects:

- Latex condoms can cause irritation in people who are allergic to latex. (True latex allergies only affect about 1% of the U.S. population but about 6% may experience symptoms of contact dermatitis such as redness, itching, or swelling after contact with latex-containing products.)

Internal (Female) Condom

The internal condom is a plastic tube-like pouch with a flexible ring at each end to help it stay in place in the vagina. It is coated inside and outside with a lubricant. The closed ring end covers the back of the vagina and cervix, the other end is open and sits at the opening to the vagina. The penis enters the vagina through the open end. The closed end prevents sperm from entering the vagina.

The internal condom can be put in place up to 8 hours before sex. After sex, you remove the condom and throw it away. Each internal condom can only be used once. You should not use internal condoms and male condoms together because they can stick to each other and cause tearing. If the condom rips or falls out of your vagina, you should consider taking emergency contraception as soon as possible within five days (see the section on EC).

Unfortunately, internal condoms can be hard to find. There is only one brand of internal condom available in the U.S. Some Planned Parenthood clinics, health centers, and family planning clinics provide them for free or at discounted cost. The method is covered by insurance plans that cover BCMs, but you'll need a prescription from your health care provider before you can buy them at your local pharmacy. You can also order them on the manufacturer's website (www.fc2.us.com) or use their site to locate an online clinician who will provide you with a prescription. A package of 12 internal condoms costs about $29; a package of 24 costs about $48. They will be mailed to your address at no additional cost.

If always used correctly, 5 out of 100 women will get pregnant each year using internal condoms. If internal condoms are not always used correctly, 21 out of 100 women will get pregnant each year.

Pros:

- The internal condom is safe, simple, and convenient.
- You can insert it ahead of time or during sex.
- The internal condom is the only birth control method controlled by the woman that also protects against most sexually transmitted infections (STIs).

- They are latex-free and made of nitrile, which, according to its manufacturer, is thinner and stronger than latex.
- They may be free at local clinics or can be purchased online.

Cons:

- You must use it every time you have sex.
- It is less effective at preventing pregnancy than some other birth control methods.
- It requires a prescription and can be hard to find in local pharmacies and clinics.
- It is more expensive than a male condom (cost is about $2 to $4 per condom), but that is cheaper than some other methods.
- The newer internal condom is said to be less "squeaky" than the original version; adding extra lubricant can help.
- Both partners will be able to see and feel the internal condom; both should be in agreement about using this method.

Side effects:

- It may cause irritation of the vagina or penis, but few studies have been done.

Liz and Josh's decision: The diaphragm

Liz is successfully using the LAM method of birth control, but as the baby gets older, she knows she'll need another method. They'd rather not use hormones while Liz is nursing the baby. For Liz and Josh, an unplanned pregnancy would be inconvenient, but would not be awful. They talk it through and conclude that they would not be bothered by using a birth control method that needs to be managed with every act of intercourse. While she liked the sponge, it was not effective enough for women who have already given birth. Still a bit unsure, Liz decides that she will make an appointment with her obstetrician/gynecologist to discuss whether to use a cervical cap or a diaphragm.

Daphne

Daphne is a 43-year-old heterosexual woman and is a single mom. She is not currently in a sexual relationship. When needed, she has used condoms for birth control, but Daphne would prefer to find a method that is 'very effective at preventing an unplanned pregnancy and something that she can control herself. She would be devastated if she became pregnant. Daphne used to have heavy painful periods, but they got better after she had Jade. She is not yet having any menopausal symptoms like hot flashes or missed periods. Since Jade started talking to Daphne about birth control, Daphne has been doing some research online to explore their options.

Daphne's priorities:

- Efficacy — how effective is the method at preventing pregnancy?
- Side effects — what kind of side effects might occur? What would I like or dislike?
- Control — do I want to rely on my partner to use the BCM or do I want to be in control?
- Protection against sexually transmitted infections — what is my risk?

[See Decision Tree #3]

Decision Tree #3: Daphne

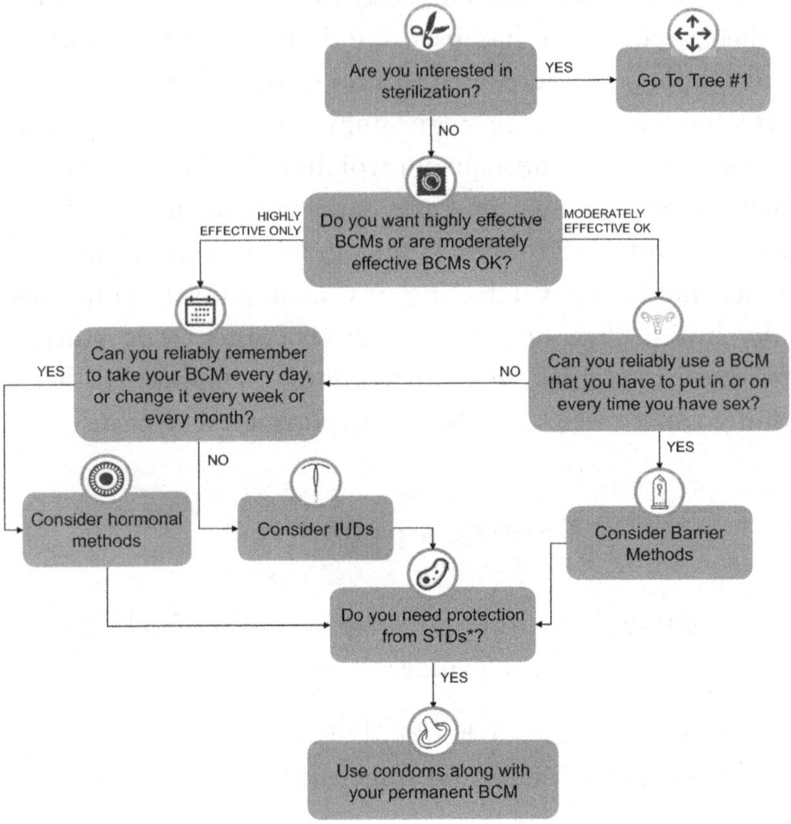

*You don't need protection from sexually transmitted diseases (STDs) if you and your partner(s) have tested STD-free and are only having sex with each other.

Daphne's options:

Sterilization and barrier methods are available to Daphne, but she is not interested in having a surgical procedure to have her tubes tied, nor is she interested in barrier methods that rely on her partner's cooperation. She wants to be in control. Daphne is most interested in the hormonal methods available.

Combination hormone-containing methods

The first hormonal method of birth control became available in the 1960s. The birth control pills contained a combination of an estrogen and a progesterone, two hormones that are naturally produced by a woman's body. In response to the additional hormones, the body reacts three ways to prevent pregnancy:

1. The body stops releasing eggs from the woman's ovaries so there is no egg for a sperm to fertilize. The eggs are reabsorbed by the body, and the woman continues to have her period.

2. The mucus in the cervix thickens, which prevents the sperm from getting into the uterus.

3. The layers of cells inside the uterus become thinner so in the rare case that an egg got fertilized, it wouldn't implant and be supported. The thinner lining is why your periods are lighter when using the pill.

Since then, millions of women have used hormonal BCMs. Today there are three methods of birth control that contain combination hormones (in much smaller amounts than in the 1960s). They are all very effective at preventing pregnancy especially if they are used correctly. Forgetting to take a pill every day, or forgetting to change your ring or patch, will put you at risk for pregnancy. Some medications can interfere with the hormones in these methods — always check with your health care provider if you are taking medication — even antibiotics — and use a condom until you can check in with them.

Individuals who have had blood clots, breast cancer, heart attacks, strokes, migraines with auras, uncontrolled high blood pressure, difficult-to-control diabetes, or liver disease may be encouraged to use alternative BCMs.

Pros:

- There are so many advantages to using estrogen-progestin combination methods, I have listed them in Table 3.

TABLE 3. ADVANTAGES OF COMBINATION HORMONAL METHODS: THE PILL, THE PATCH, THE VAGINAL RING	
Improved	Menstrual control — you can use the pills to alter the timing of your periods or use them continuously to prevent your periods, at no harm to you
Reduced	Symptoms of menstrual migraine with extended cycle or continuous estrogen-progestin contraception
	Dysmenorrhea (painful periods, menstrual cramps)
	Irregular menstrual cycles
	Pelvic pain related to endometriosis
	Menorrhagia (heavy periods)
	Iron-deficiency anemia related to menstrual blood loss
	Risk of ectopic pregnancy
	Risk of pelvic inflammatory disease (PID)
	Symptoms associated with premenstrual syndrome (PMS) like headaches, irritability, and depression

TABLE 3. ADVANTAGES OF COMBINATION HORMONAL METHODS: THE PILL, THE PATCH, THE VAGINAL RING	
Reduced	Risk of benign breast disease
	Development of ovarian cysts (higher-dose pills only), no effect on existing cysts
	Risk of ovarian cancer, including those associated with mutations in the BRCA1 or BRCA2 gene
	Endometrial (uterine) cancer
	Colorectal cancer in current users
	Moderate acne
	Hirsutism (unwanted hair growth)
	Postmenopausal hip fracture risk for women who use estrogen-containing contraceptives in their 40s
	Acne and vasomotor symptoms (hot flashes) in perimenopausal women

Cons:

- If you use the pill, the patch, or the ring, you need to be very careful about your schedule. You need to be able to take the pill at the same time every day, change the patch once a week, or insert a new ring every three to four weeks. You need to have enough supplies on hand so that you don't run out.

- Not everyone can use combination hormone-containing methods If you are over 35 years old and smoke, you should not use these methods. If you have had heart, liver, or blood clotting issues, lupus, migraines with auras, high blood pressure, or some other conditions, these methods are not for you. If you have, or have had, medical issues, talk to your health care provider so you can choose a method that is the safest and most effective one for you.

- They provide no protection from STIs.

- Some medicines can interfere with the hormones in the pill, the ring, and the patch — consult your health care provider if you are taking medicine and want to use hormonal methods.

Side effects:

- Headaches, nausea, tender breasts, or light bleeding between periods (spotting) can occur when you first start using hormonal BCMs. Normally, they go away once your body gets used to the method, usually after 2 or 3 months.

- Lighter than normal periods or cessation of periods — neither of these cause harm to your body. If you don't like these side effects, other methods are available to you.

- Heart attack, stroke, blood clots, or liver tumor, any of which can cause death. All of these occur very rarely.

- Some women report mood changes, depression or anxiety that may start or worsen when using hormonal products. Consult a health care professional.

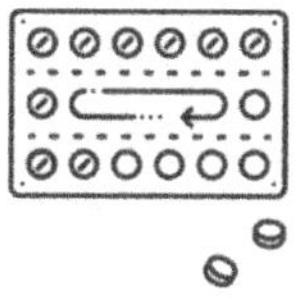

Oral Contraceptives ("the Pill")

There are many brands of birth control pills available. They all must be taken every day at the same time. As of today, they require a prescription from your health care provider. (But there are advocates working to make the pills available over-the-counter, like they are in many countries. Check in with freethepill.org for more information.)

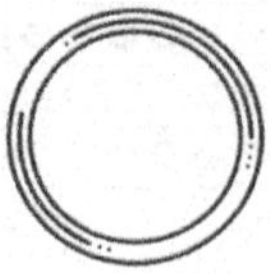

Vaginal Ring

The vaginal ring is a thin, flexible plastic ring that you place in the back of your vagina. It releases small amounts of the two hormones, estrogen and progesterone. After three to five weeks you remove it, wait a week (during which time you will have a period) and then replace it with another one. If you don't want to have a period, you can change it every three to five weeks with no time off.

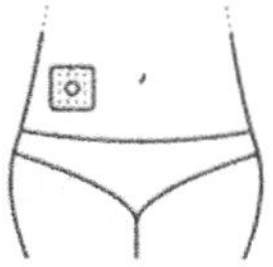

Skin Patch

The "Patch" looks like a thin, square adhesive Band-Aid that you place on your abdomen or arm. It releases the hormones estrogen and progesterone, which are absorbed by the skin. You change the patch once a week for 3 weeks then take a week off. If you want to skip your period you can use the patch continuously. Your period will return when you stop using the patch for a few days.

Progestin-only hormonal methods

Progestin-only methods, like combination hormonal products, work by preventing the ovaries from releasing an egg, thicken the mucus in the cervix to block the sperm from entering the uterus, and may rarely prevent a fertilized egg from implanting in the uterus. These methods include progestin-only pills (also called mini-pills), the injection or shot, implants, and IUDs.

Pros:

- Do not affect breast milk supply
- Reduce heavy menstrual bleeding and cramping
- Can be used short term or long term; can be stopped at any time
- Do not interfere with sexual spontaneity
- Can be used by women who cannot take estrogen — like smokers older than 35, women with heart disease, blood clots, high blood pressure, anemia, sickle cell disease, poorly controlled diabetes, or migraines with auras

Cons:

- Pills must be taken at the same time every day

Side effects:

- Irregular periods or spotting or bleeding between periods
- Amenorrhea (no menstrual periods) — more likely with the shot and the hormonal IUD
- Sore breasts, nausea, headache, bloating — these usually go away after a few cycles
- Weight gain — more likely with the shot than other progestin-only methods
- Depression — rarely
- Darkening of the skin on areas of the face — rarely
- Higher risk of developing diabetes in women who had gestational diabetes (diabetes that occurs during pregnancy) — rarely

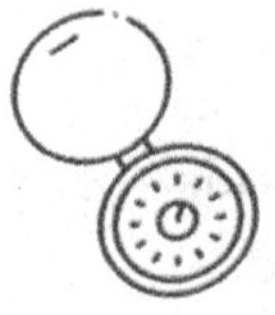

Progestin-only Pills (Mini-pills)

Mini-pills that contain only progesterone are not quite as effective as combination oral contraceptives that contain both estrogen and progesterone. So it is very important to take the progestin-only pills at the same time every day. If you miss a pill you should use an extra method of birth control for the next few days. If you recently had sex and had forgotten to take a pill, you should consider using emergency contraception (see the section on EC). Nausea, vomiting, and some medications may interfere with the effectiveness of the mini-pill. Always ask your health care provider when starting any new medication. Have a backup method of birth control ready — condoms are easy to have on hand.

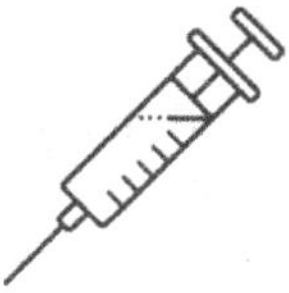

Birth Control Injection (the Shot)

The birth control shot contains progesterone and is injected into the upper arm or buttock every three months. It is effective right away if it is given within five days of your last menstrual period. It is a very effective method of birth control.

Things to consider:

- It should not be used by women who have unexplained vaginal bleeding or those who have had breast cancer, liver disease, or blood clots.
- Many women experience changes in their menstrual periods, like spotting or irregular bleeding, when using the injection for birth control. After a year of use, about 50% of women will stop getting their periods. Their periods usually return quickly when they stop getting the shots. Not having your period

is not harmful to your body, though its effect on bone density over many years needs more study.

- Although you can get pregnant within three or four months after your last injection, it can take some women more than a year to get pregnant. It doesn't seem to matter how long you have used it for this to occur.
- Using the shot every three months for over two years may cause a decrease in the density of your bones, so talk to your health care provider if you may want to use it for longer than that period of time.
- Women with sickle cell disease may have fewer problems from their disease when using the birth control shot, so this would be a good method for them.

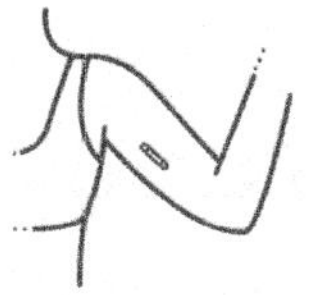

Hormonal Rod Implants

The implant is a small plastic rod about the size of a matchstick that contains progesterone. The skin of your upper arm is numbed and then the rod is inserted under the skin by your health care provider. This is done in the office or clinic and takes less than a minute. You'll be able to feel the rod under your skin but you won't be able to see it.

The implant is one of only a few long-acting reversible contraceptive (LARC) methods (the others are the injection and IUDs). One rod lasts for three years or more before it needs to be replaced. It can be easily removed at any time if you decide you want to get pregnant. Because it lasts for at least three years, the cost of the implant is one of the cheaper methods of birth control.

Daphne's decision:
The vaginal ring

Because Daphne is not currently in a sexual relationship, she wants a BCM that is available when she needs it but not something that is affecting her body all the time. She also wants a method that is discreet and is concerned that barrier methods are not as effective as she'd like. Daphne was very interested in the combination hormone methods when she saw the list of benefits, but she is over 35 so has an increased risk of side effects from estrogen. She is also concerned about having to consistently take a pill at the same time every day. She is afraid she might mess up now and then. So, Daphne decides that she is most interested in the patch or the vaginal ring. When Daphne learns that the vaginal ring is used by some women to decrease menopausal symptoms like hot flashes and that it has one of the highest satisfaction rates among users, she is convinced that this is the right method for her now.[9]

Jade

Jade is 18 years old and has a boyfriend she has been with for about a year. So far, they have been practicing abstinence. But Jade felt that abstinence was not realistic. She and her boyfriend had been exploring sexual activities like dry humping and mutual masturbation but have not had oral, vaginal, or anal intercourse. Jade's boyfriend had purchased condoms to have just in case.

Jade felt strongly that not using a BCM would be irresponsible. She did not want to have a child or an abortion and she knew that effective BCMs are readily available and affordable. She was looking forward to the time when she and a partner were ready to become sexually active, and she wanted that experience to be free from concern about the possibility of getting pregnant or contracting a sexually transmitted infection. She was prepared to use condoms to prevent an STI and was ready to choose the method of birth control that would best prevent an unwanted pregnancy.

Jade has a good relationship with her mom and has talked to her about sex and birth control. Jade will be leaving for college soon and thinks she should start a birth control method so that if she becomes sexually active, she will be ready. Daphne, Jade's mom, thinks this a very good idea, but isn't sure how to advise her daughter. Together, they search some internet sites to get more information about what Jade should use. (See the Resources section for a list of this book for a list of recommended sites.)

Jade's priorities:

- Impact — how would an unplanned pregnancy affect my life? Could I handle having a baby or an abortion?
- Efficacy — how effective is the method at preventing pregnancy?
- Convenience — how easy is the method to use?
- Side effects — what can I put up with in order to prevent pregnancy?
- Control — do I want to rely on my partner to use the BCM or do I want to be in control?
- Protection against sexually transmitted infections — what is my risk?

[See Decision Tree #3]

Jade's options:

All methods of birth control are available to Jade. Here we'll cover the methods we haven't talked about yet.

Abstinence

To some people, abstinence means not participating in any sexual activities at all. To others, abstinence means not having penis-in-vagina intercourse, but all other sexual activities are permitted. Regardless of what your definition is, abstinence can be a very effective way to prevent pregnancy as long as semen does not come in contact with a vagina. Some individuals use abstinence before they decide to be sexually active, others use it between sexual partners, and others live a complete, healthy life without ever having sexual intercourse at all. Some, but not all, religions advocate for the practice of abstinence unless a couple is married. The choice is yours.

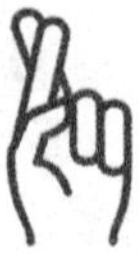

No Birth Control Method

Once an individual decides to participate in sexual activity that includes male semen near female genitals, pregnancy is a potential outcome. If pregnancy is a desired outcome, then BCMs are not necessary. Without the use of a BCM, 85 out of 100 sexually active heterosexual women will become pregnant within one year.

Pros:

- No hormones, devices, or injections
- No cost

Cons:

- No protection from pregnancy
- No protection from STIs

Side effects:

- Worry about pregnancy

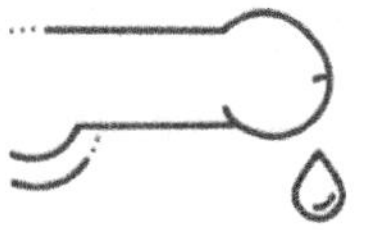

Withdrawal

This method requires that the man remove his penis from the woman's vagina before he ejaculates. As this is hard to control, it is difficult to do correctly with every act of intercourse. In addition, sperm reside in pre-ejaculation fluid, so there is risk of pregnancy prior to ejaculation. However, the method is free and always available with no side effects. It may be used by couples who follow religious rules against using contraception, though 89% to 90% of Catholic and Protestant women at risk of getting pregnant use a BCM.[10] Withdrawal is less effective for men with less sexual experience and for those under the influence of alcohol or drugs. Couples who are sexually experienced and are committed to using this method can use it successfully. However, in general use, it is less effective than other BCMs.

Pros:

- No hormones, devices, or injections
- No cost

Cons:

- Not highly effective (due to the difficulty of controlling timing of ejaculation)
- Little protection from STIs
- Requires male partners to be highly motivated

Side effects:

- Worry about pregnancy

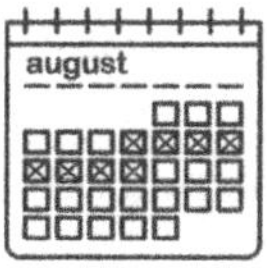

Fertility Awareness or Natural Family Planning (Rhythm Method)

This method of birth control requires that the woman carefully monitors her menstrual cycle using signs like her daily temperature and changes in her cervical mucus to predict when in her menstrual cycle she is most likely to ovulate. The couple either refrains from sex during the fertile interval (usually 2 weeks mid-cycle) or uses a condom or other barrier method during that time. This method is best used by women with regular periods and by couples who are very devoted to natural family planning. There are many books that provide detailed descriptions of the various ways to use this method. In general use, approximately 24 out of every 100 couples using this method will get pregnant within one year.

Pros:

- Can be very effective if used correctly and consistently

- No hormones, devices, or injections
- Increased awareness of natural hormonal cycles
- Little, if any, cost

Cons:

- Not highly effective due to difficulty of perfect use
- No protection from STIs except when condoms are used
- Requires both partners to be highly motivated
- Not effective for women with irregular cycles

Side effects:

- None

Intrauterine devices (IUDs)

IUDs, implants, and the injection are called LARCs (long-acting reversible contraception). These are the most effective non-permanent methods of birth control available today. Once they are inserted or injected you don't have to think about birth control again for months or years! No pills to remember to take, nothing to put in or on you right before sex, nothing to remember to take with you. They do not protect against STIs though, so if you are at risk, you still have to remember your condoms!

IUDs have been in use since the 1960s and, like the pill, have improved over the years. The two IUDs discussed below can be used by most women including teenagers and women over 35, women who have had babies and those who have not, and women with medical conditions that preclude them from using combination hormonal contraception.

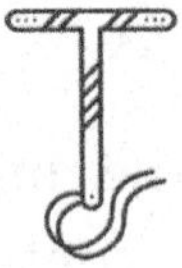

Copper IUD

The copper IUD is one of two types of intrauterine devices available in the U.S. The other type is the hormone-containing IUD (see the next section). Today's IUDs are smaller, safer, and more effective than those used in the 1970s. The copper IUD is a small, flexible device made of soft plastic wound with thin copper wire. It is easily inserted into the uterus by a health care provider at an office visit. It effectively prevents pregnancy as soon as it is inserted.

Copper ions that escape from the thin copper wire thicken the mucus in the cervix, preventing the sperm from getting into the uterus. The copper ions also inhibit the movement of any sperm that do get in, and they may make the uterine walls inhospitable to a fertilized egg, preventing implantation.

A copper IUD can also be inserted up to five days after unprotected sex as emergency contraception to prevent pregnancy, then kept in place to provide ongoing birth control.

The copper IUD is one of the most effective birth control methods available. Fewer than 1 out of

1000 women who use it will get pregnant each year.[11] This is as effective as a tubal ligation — but unlike sterilization, you can become pregnant quickly once the IUD is removed.

Pros:

- It is highly effective at preventing pregnancy.
- It lowers your risk for cervical cancer.[12]
- It can last up to 12 years before it needs to be removed and replaced with a new one.
- It does not contain hormones or interact with medicines.
- You don't have to think about birth control every day or every time you have sex.
- You can have the IUD easily removed at any time and your fertility quickly returns to normal.
- Because one IUD can be used for so long, it is one of the least expensive methods of birth control.

Cons:

- It does not protect against sexually transmitted infections (STIs).
- You must visit your health care provider to have it inserted and removed.
- The initial cost is high if not covered by insurance.
- If you become pregnant with an IUD in place (very rare), you are at higher risk for miscarriage, pre-term delivery, and uterine infections.

Side effects:

- You may have more bleeding and cramping with your periods at first, but this usually lessens over time.
- It is possible for the IUD to slip out of place, but this is rare.
- It can get stuck in or puncture the uterus during insertion and will need to be removed, but this happens very rarely.

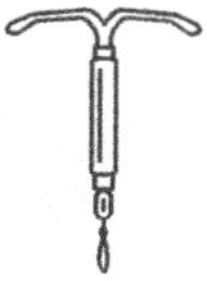

Hormonal IUDs

The hormonal IUD contains progesterone, is highly effective, and can be inserted into your uterus at any time. The procedure is done in the health care provider's office or clinic and takes only a few minutes. You may experience mild cramping and light bleeding or spotting for one or two days. It is effective immediately. Depending on which brand you use, it is effective for three to seven years before it needs to be replaced. Several brands are available on the U.S. market.

Getting pregnant with an IUD in place is very rare. Most pregnancies happen because the IUD gets pushed out of (expelled from) the uterus unnoticed. This is most likely to occur within the first few months of getting an IUD, or if it was inserted just after childbirth. You can check by feeling for the string of your IUD to be sure it hasn't been expelled. You should be able to feel a very thin plastic string coming out from the dimple in your cervix at the back of your vagina. Your health care provider will teach you how to do this.

Pros:

- It is highly effective at preventing pregnancy.
- It can last from three to seven years before it needs to be removed and replaced with a new one.
- Reduces heavy menstrual bleeding and cramps after the first few months.
- May eventually cause your period to stop altogether, which is not harmful.
- May prevent endometrial hyperplasia and endometrial cancer, and relieve endometriosis.
- Reduces the risk of ectopic pregnancy.
- Does not cause weight gain.

Cons:

- It does not protect against sexually transmitted infections (STIs).
- You must visit your health care provider to have it inserted and removed.
- Even though it is not harmful, you may be uncomfortable not having your period. If your periods stop altogether, you may worry about being pregnant.

- The initial cost is high if not covered by insurance.

Side effects:

- It may cause ovarian cysts, which usually go away on their own.
- It can have other hormone-related side effects, including spotting, mood swings, and breast tenderness, but these occur less frequently than with other progestin-only methods.
- It can get stuck in or puncture the uterus during insertion and will need to be removed, but this happens very rarely.

Jade's decision: The copper IUD

Jade and Daphne find a lot of information about birth control methods on the internet. They are surprised to find that most adolescents and young adults have used short-acting contraceptive methods (condoms, the pill, the patch, the vaginal ring, and the shot) that have lower continuation rates and higher pregnancy rates than long-acting reversible contraceptive (LARC) methods (IUDs and the implant). Studies have found that complications from using IUDs and implants are rare and that adolescents are at no higher risk than older women. The American Academy of Pediatrics states that LARCs "are the best reversible methods for preventing unintended pregnancy, repeat pregnancies, and abortion in young women."[13]

Jade doesn't like the idea that she would have to go to a clinic, doctor's office, or pharmacy every few months or so to get supplies — especially when she is away from home. She likes how effective the IUD is and how she will not have to worry about pregnancy or birth control for years. But when, and if, she decides she is ready to have a child, she can have it removed and get pregnant right away. She likes that the hormone-containing IUD would lessen her periods and cramping, but she doesn't like the idea of not having a period at all. And she likes that the copper IUD has no hormones and lasts over 10 years. But she is concerned about the cost. Daphne tells her that she thinks their health insurancc will cover it. They figure out that the IUD is one of the cheapest methods of birth control when you consider how long it lasts. Jade feels happy that she has made a responsible decision about her body and her future. She and her mom are both comfortable with their decisions and pleased that they do not have to worry about an unplanned pregnancy.

Daniella

Daniella is a 17-year-old transgender woman. She was born with male genitalia and was designated male at birth. But Daniella never felt like she was a boy. This was not much of a problem for her as a child but around middle-school she started to feel pressure to be more boy-like by boys and girls and adults alike. Her innate desires were to become more girl-like but that wasn't happening socially or within her own body. It was a very confusing time for her.

Daniella's mother was more accepting of her than her father, but Daniella felt she was adding stress to an already stressed family situation. When Jade, after consulting with Daphne, asked Daniella if she wanted to stay at her house for a while, everyone agreed. In a safer environment, Daniella has been able to explore her gender identity and experiment with her gender expression. She is feeling more confident in herself now.

After consulting a health care provider, Daniella began taking gender-affirming hormone therapy a few years ago. She is aware that while the estrogen she takes will decrease the number of sperm that develop, her sperm count is not lowered enough to depend on for birth control. She also worries that taking estrogen may affect her long-term fertility, but knows that her health care provider is monitoring that at the clinic she attends.

Daniella joined Jade and Daphne in their online search for the birth control method that would be the best choice for each of them.

Daniella's priorities:

- Do I want kids someday? — Should I choose a permanent or a temporary method? Am I sure about my decision to have or not have children?
- Impact — how would an unplanned pregnancy affect my life? Could I handle having a baby?
- Side effects — What kinds of unwanted side effects might occur? What can I put up with in order to prevent pregnancy? Could there be side effects I would like?
- Control — do I want to rely on my partner to use the BCM or do I want to be in control?
- Protection against sexually transmitted infections — what is my risk?

[See Decision Tree #3]

Daniella's options:

Following their research, Daniella concluded that men and transwomen have many fewer contraceptive options than do cisgender women. Basically, she is limited to abstinence, withdrawal, male condoms and permanent options like vasectomy. (See abstinence, withdrawal, male condoms and vasectomy sections above.)

In her search, Daniella learned that several methods of male contraception are currently being evaluated in studies including: a male birth control pill and a male injection both based on a hormone or a hormone and steroid combination, a birth control gel that is rubbed into the skin daily, a gel injected into the vas deferens as a kind of reversable vasectomy, and a less-invasive vasectomy technique using a puncture, rather than an incision in the scrotum.[14] None of these methods are close to being approved, but Daniella was happy to know they are in the contraceptive pipeline.

Daniella's decision: Abstinence

Daniella is not sexually involved with anyone at this time. Her past relationships have not escalated to the point of having genital sex. For now, Daniella will continue to use abstinence but she is happy to know about all the methods of birth control and how they work.

Daniella decides that if she would become involved in a sexual relationship with a person of any gender, male condoms would protect them both from STIs. They are easy to use, cheap, and always available, so Daniella decides to buy some to keep on-hand.

Depending on whether or not she wants children someday, she may consider a permanent method like a vasectomy, but she doesn't feel ready to make that decision yet.

Emergency Contraception (EC)

Emergency contraception is NOT a form of birth control. EC is useful for episodes of unplanned unprotected intercourse. Accidents can happen. Emergency contraception is available if:

- you weren't using any birth control when you had sex,
- you forgot to take your birth control pills, or change your patch, ring, or other birth control method,
- your or your partner's condom broke or slipped off,
- your partner didn't pull out in time,
- you were forced to have unprotected vaginal sex.[15]

Some form of emergency contraception is now available in the U.S. and many other countries to individuals of any age without a prescription. (See Table 4.) There are two methods available to prevent conception after an unprotected act of intercourse: hormonal pills or an IUD. Many individuals will keep the over-the-counter (OTC) pills or a prescription for the prescription-only pills on hand in case they need to use them someday.

Hormonal pills for EC

Also known as morning-after pills, the sooner after sex you take them, the more effective they are. There are three formulations of pills available in pharmacies.

1. Levonorgestrel-containing pills (1.5 mg in a single dose) are available OTC without a prescription. There are several brand names including Plan B One-Step, which is available to individuals regardless of gender without age restrictions. Other brands are available OTC to individuals regardless of gender who are 17 years of age or older. These pills are effective when taken within the first 3 days after unprotected sex. They are not effective when taken later. It is estimated that 87 out of 100 women who would have become pregnant will not become pregnant after taking these pills.[16]

2. Ulipristal-containing pills (30 mg in a single dose) are only available with a prescription from a health care provider. The brand name is ella. There are no age restrictions. Of all the oral contraceptive pills, ella is the most effective. It must be taken within 5 days of unprotected vaginal intercourse. It is estimated that 94 or 95 out of every 100 women who would have become pregnant will not become pregnant after taking ella.[10]

3. Combination estrogen-progestin-containing pills (2 pills at one time followed by 2 more pills 12 hours later). Most of the birth control pills on the market contain a combination of estrogen and progesterone (except for progesterone-only pills). They must be taken within 3 days of unprotected vaginal intercourse to prevent pregnancy and are not effective when taken after that timeframe. It is estimated that 75 out of 100 women who would have become pregnant will not become pregnant after taking the combination birth control pills in this manner.

Copper IUD for EC

The copper IUD is the most effective method available for preventing an unwanted pregnancy if it is inserted within 5 days of unprotected intercourse. (See Copper IUD section for a description)

The biggest advantage of using this method of emergency contraception is that you will never need emergency contraception again! The IUD can be kept in your uterus for up to 12 years before it needs to be replaced. You can get pregnant immediately after removal of the IUD. If you are overweight, the IUD is most effective.

Pros:

- The benefits of taking EC outweigh the potential side effects, so most women can use EC without restriction.
- All forms of EC are very effective. The copper IUD is the most effective, followed by ella, then the levonorgestrel-containing pills, followed by the combined hormonal pills.
- All forms of EC are readily available in the event of an unplanned episode of unprotected intercourse. Hormonal pills are the most readily available and may be kept in your home in case they are needed.

The levonorgestrel-containing pills are available over-the-counter (without a prescription) in U.S. pharmacies.

- All forms of EC are private. No one else has to know you have taken or used it. The copper IUD and ella both require a prescription.
- Once the copper IUD is inserted, it can be used as your regular form of birth control for up to 12 years until it needs to be replaced. The copper IUD is as effective as a tubal ligation or vasectomy.
- The IUD, the levonorgesterone pills and ella can be used by smokers, people over 35, and nursing mothers since they do not contain estrogen.

Cons:

- Some forms of EC require a prescription or office visit (ella and IUD).
- EC methods do not work beyond their effectiveness timelines (3 to 5 days depending on method). If a woman is already pregnant, EC methods will not work.
- EC methods do not protect against STIs. If you are concerned about potential STIs following your unprotected intercourse, get tested.

Side effects:

- EC pills may cause nausea, vomiting, stomach pain, or headaches, most of which are temporary (many resolve within 24 hours) and not serious. There are no known long-term side-effects.
- The copper IUD can cause pain and cramping during insertion and may cause a heavier than normal period.

TABLE 4. EMERGENCY CONTRACEPTIVE METHODS*

Emergency contraception	Levonorgestrel-containing pill	Ulipristal-containing pill	Copper IUD
Effectiveness:	Good	Better	Best
When to use it:	Up to 3 to 5 days after unprotected sex	Up to 5 days after unprotected sex	Up to 5 days after unprotected sex
Use with caution if:	Overweight or obese (less effective)	Breastfeeding (should not use), obese (less effective)	Serious allergy to copper or deformed uterus (both are rare)
Availability:	Without a prescription at pharmacy or clinic	By prescription at pharmacy or clinic	At your health care provider's office or clinic
Contraceptive effect:	Does not prevent pregnancy from sex you have after you take it	Does not prevent pregnancy from sex you have after you take it	Continues to prevent pregnancy for 12 years

* Adapted from http://www.plannedparenthood.org/health-info/morning-after-pill-emergency-contraception

The Cost of Birth Control

Effective birth control methods save money — for individuals and for society. Consider the medical costs for prenatal care and birth and then add in the costs of raising a child (estimated to be from $13,000 to $15,000 per year per child).[17] Even the most expensive form of birth control does not come close to the cost of having one child. Contraception saves money by reducing unintended pregnancies and reducing transmission of sexually transmitted infections (STIs), too. Not using contraception is the most expensive option.

The most effective and the most cost-effective methods are long-acting methods like implants, IUDs, and sterilization. But the up-front cost of these methods have prevented some women from using them.[18] When the Affordable Care Act was passed in 2010, all contraceptive methods approved in the U.S. were listed as essential health care to be covered by health insurance plans. Some religious organizations objected to providing coverage for BCMs and were successful in removing the mandated coverage from the legislation. Now, unless your health plan is sponsored by certain religious employers, your birth control method should be available to you at no additional out-of-pocket costs or co-pays. This includes emergency contraception. Even over-the-counter birth control may be covered, but you might need to show a prescription from a health care provider. If you have insurance, check with a plan representative to see if your BCM method is covered. If you do not have coverage and can't afford to pay for it, many clinics and health departments provide BCMs on a sliding scale fee and some methods, like condoms, may be free.

Choosing *Your* Birth Control Method

As we have seen, the women in the Miller family had many things to think about before they made their decisions. The first thing they did was to gather information about the birth control methods that are available. This is important because progress is always being made to improve and increase the number of contraceptive options. Check the Resources section for a list of some reliable sources of information about birth control that you can refer to when making your own decision.

To help you, I have designed a worksheet (see Appendix II) that you can use to narrow down your options. Using the worksheet along with this manual should help you make your decision about what method is the right one for you at this time in your life. Another good resource is on the Planned Parenthood website at: http://www.plannedparenthood.org/all-access/my-method

Before we are finished, I have a few more words of advice.

Recommendation #3:
You can always change your birth control method, but try using it for at least three to six months before deciding you don't like it.

When starting a new BCM, it may take some time before you are comfortable using it, especially if it is a method that you need to learn how to track, insert, put on, or change periodically. As with all new things, it takes a little time to get used to. If you experience side effects from your BCM that are severe or unexpected, call or visit your health care provider for advice. Check out the expected side effects of your new BCM in this book or online to see if they are common. Many side effects go away completely or become less bothersome over time. If, at the end of three to six months, you are still uncomfortable with the symptoms you are experiencing, you can always change your method. It is nice to know that you now have many options to choose from — and you don't need to rely on lambskins and herbs to control your fertility!

Recommendation #4:
Your health care provider is your friend.

Find a clinic, a physician, or a nurse practitioner with whom you feel comfortable discussing your birth control needs. These health care providers are highly trained experts who discuss these matters with patients every day.

While you may feel a bit awkward discussing personal issues, they will not — that's their job. Especially if you are having any problems with your BCM, if you are having trouble paying for your BCM, or if you have any symptoms of an STI (burning, irritation, discharge, odor, pain), contact them quickly to resolve the problem. They are there to help you.

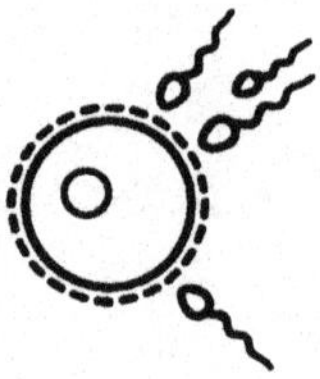

Resources

- **Advocates for Youth**
  Including youth partners in advocacy and education
  https://advocatesforyouth.org/

- **American Sexual Health Association**
  Resources on sexual health for men and women
  www.ashasexualhealth.org

- **Association of Reproductive Health Professionals (ARHP)**
  www.arhp.org

- **Bedsider**
  Online BCM support network for young women
  http://bedsider.org/

- **Birth control methods**
  https://www.fda.gov/consumers/free-publications-women/birth-control

- **Condomania**
  A source for condoms, sex toys, lubricants and other such items.
  Condomania.com

- **Emergency contraception**

  - https://www.hhs.gov/opa/pregnancy-prevention/birth-control-methods/emergency-contraception/index.html

  - https://www.womenshealth.gov/a-z-topics/emergency-contraception

- **Free the Pill**
  Efforts to make the birth control pill available over the counter (OTC)
  www.freethepill.org

- **Get Tested**
  Find free, confidential STI testing near you
  Gettested.cdc.gov

- **LGBT Youth Resources**
  Resources for LGBT youth and friends/supporters
  www.cdc.gov/lgbthealth/youth-resources.htm

- **My Pill app**
  Get refills, reminders to take pills, etc.
  www.mypillapp.com

- **Office of Women's Health**
  U.S. Department of Health and Human Services
  Birth control method information
  http://womenshealth.gov/publications/our-publications/fact-sheet/birth-control-methods.html?from=AtoZ

- **Planned Parenthood**
  Online tools for questions about BCMs, STI testing
  http://www.plannedparenthood.org/all-access/my-method

- **Planned Parenthood Direct app**
  Online access to birth control methods, on-line clinician interactions, treatment for urinary tract infections, help finding a health center
  https://plannedparenthooddirect.org/

- **Sexplanations**
  Dr. Lindsey Doe inspires curiosity and explains things
  Youtube.com/sexplanations.

- **Web MD**
  Compare birth control methods
  www.webmd.com/a-to-z-guides/effectiveness-rate-of-birth-control-methods-topic-overview

Appendix I: Birth Control Method Chart

Method	Description	How it Works	Side Effects	Number of unplanned pregnancies out of 100 typical users
No birth control	No barrier to sperm entering the cervix and fertilizing an egg	It doesn't	None	85
Abstinence	Sexual activity that does not include genital contact	Prevents sperm from entering the cervix	None	0 if used perfectly
With-drawal	The man removes his penis from the woman's vagina before he ejaculates.	Prevents sperm from entering the vagina	None	4 if used perfect-ly, 27 if not
Natural Family Planning/ Fertility Awareness/ Rhythm Method	Refraining from sex during the more fertile times of a woman's menstrual cycle as determined by close moni-toring of cycle each month	Prevents sperm from entering the cervix during a woman's more fertile time	None	24 due to diffi-culty of perfect use

Protection from STIs?	Prescription-only (Rx) or Over-the-counter (OTC)	Discreet	Interval of Use	Cost*	Who should use it? Anyone who:	Who should NOT use it? Anyone who:
No	NA	No	Never	No cost	Doesn't mind if they get pregnant	Wants to prevent getting pregnant
Yes	NA	No	Daily		Is sure they won't have intercourse	Might have unplanned intercourse
No	NA	No	Every act of intercourse		Can consistently withdraw prior to ejaculation	Cannot consistently withdraw or are under influence of alcohol or drugs
No	NA	No	Daily		Is highly motivated, has a regular menstrual cycle. May use barrier method during fertile times.	Cannot consistently monitor their cycle or who has a partner who does not agree or commit to method

BARRIER METHODS				
Method	Description	How it Works	Side Effects	Number of unplanned pregnancies out of 100 typical users
Sponge (Today®), Cervical Cap	Small circular sponge or fitted silicone cup inserted into the vagina to cover the cervix. They contain or are used with spermicide.	Blocks sperm from entering cervix; disables sperm from being able to fertilize an egg	Slightly elevated risk of vaginosis, yeast infection, toxic shock syndrome if left in place over 24-30 hours	16 if no previous children, 32 if had child-birth
Diaphragm	A flexible latex cover for the cervix and back of the vagina. Used with spermicide. The right size is determined by clinician examinaton.	Blocks sperm from entering cervix; disables sperm from being able to fertilize an egg	Increased risk of UTI, vaginosis and yeast infection in some women	6 if used perfectly, 12 if not

BARRIER METHODS						
Protection from STIs?	Prescription-only (Rx) or Over-the-counter (OTC)	Discreet	Interval of Use	Cost*	Who should use it? Anyone who:	Who should NOT use it? Anyone who:
No	Sponge is OTC, Cap is fitted by HCP	No	Every time	Sponge: $15 for 3; Cap: $35 to $60 plus office visit, lasts 3 years	Is comfortable inserting these methods into their vagina. Anyone who wants to, or has to, avoid taking hormones.	Can't plan ahead or use the method correctly every time
No	Needs to be fitted by HCP	No	Every time	$35 to $75 plus office visit cost, lasts 3 years		

BARRIER METHODS				
Method	Description	How it Works	Side Effects	Number of unplanned pregnancies out of 100 typical users
Internal (female) Condom	A very thin plastic-like sheath with a covered ring on one end and an open ring on the other that covers the cervix and walls of the vagina and catches semen to prevent it from entering the cervix	Blocks sperm from entering cervix	None	5 if used perfectly, 21 if not
Male Condom	A thin sheath that fits over the erect penis and catches semen to prevent it from entering the cervix	Blocks sperm from entering cervix	None	2 if used perfectly, 18 if not

BARRIER METHODS						
Protection from STIs?	Prescription-only (Rx) or Over-the-counter (OTC)	Discreet	Interval of Use	Cost*	Who should use it? Anyone who:	Who should NOT use it? Anyone who:
Yes	OTC	No	Every time	$4 apiece	Is comfortable with touching their genitals. Good protection against sexually transmitted infections. Can be used with other methods for protection from STIs.	Can't plan ahead or use the method correctly every time
Yes	OTC	No	Every time	$0 to $2 apiece		

HORMONAL METHODS				
Method	Description	How it Works	Side Effects	Number of unplanned pregnancies out of 100 typical users
Combined Oral Contraceptives, "the Pill"	Estrogen and progestin-containing pills that change the woman's sex hormones and reproductive organs to prevent release of an egg, fertilization of an egg by sperm, or implantation of a fertilized egg in the uterus	Prevents ovulation or fertilization or implantation	Spotting, breast tenderness and bloating that may decrease over time. Decreased menstrual flow and cramps. Protects against ectopic pregnancy, uterine and ovarian cancer, and pelvic inflammatory disease. Reduces acne.	1 if used perfectly, 9 if not
The Patch (Ortho Evra)	Adhesive patch worn on abdomen or arm that releases estrogen and progestin	Prevents ovulation or fertilization or implantation	Similar to the Pill, skin irritation	1 if used perfectly, 9 if not

HORMONAL METHODS						
Protection from STIs?	Prescription-only (Rx) or Over-the-counter (OTC)	Discreet	Interval of Use	Cost*	Who should use it? Anyone who:	Who should NOT use it? Anyone who:
No	Rx	Yes	Daily	$15 to $50 per month	Wants a very effective but temporary method. Can remember to take a pill every day. Reduces acne and vasomotor symptoms in peri-menopausal women.	Can't take a pill every day without missing some. Smokers over 35 years old, women who have had blood clots, certain cancers and other diseases or cardiovascular risks. Discuss with clinician.
No	Rx	Maybe; can be seen on body	Change every week	$15 to $50 per month	Wants a very effective temporary method and can remember to apply a new one every week. Reduces acne and vasomotor symptoms in peri-menopausal women.	Smokes and is over 35 years old, women who have had blood clots, certain cancers and other diseases or cardiovascular risks. Discuss with clinician.

HORMONAL METHODS				
Method	Description	How it Works	Side Effects	Number of unplanned pregnancies out of 100 typical users
Vaginal Ring (Nuva Ring®)	Flexible transparent ring placed in the vagina that releases estrogen and progestin	Prevents ovulation or fertilization or implantation	Similar to the Pill, rarely vaginal discharge	1 if used perfectly, 9 if not
Progestin -only Oral Contraceptives, "Mini-pills"	Progestin-containing pills	Prevents the release of an egg and thickens the cervical mucus to prevent the passage of sperm into the uterus and may prevent the release of an egg from the ovaries	Spotting between periods, amenorrhea, tender breasts, headaches, dizziness. Protection from uterine and ovarian cancer, and PID	8

HORMONAL METHODS						
Protection from STIs?	Prescription-only (Rx) or Over-the-counter (OTC)	Discreet	Interval of Use	Cost*	Who should use it? Anyone who:	Who should NOT use it? Anyone who:
No	Rx	Maybe; may rarely be felt in vagina	Change every 3 to 4 weeks	$0 to $80 per month	Wants a very effective temporary method and can remember to apply a new patch every 3 to 4 weeks. Reduces acne and vasomotor symptoms in peri-menopausal women.	Is uncomfortable inserting the ring into their vagina. Smokers over 35 years old, women who have had blood clots, certain cancers and other diseases or cardiovascular risks. Discuss with clinician.
No	Rx	Yes	Daily	$15 to $50 per month	Wants very effective temporary method that does not contain estrogen; smokers, breastfeeding women, and women over 35	Cannot remember to take a pill at the same time every day. Anyone with current breast cancer, cardiovascular disease, lupus, migraines with aura, or other medical conditions, consult a clinician.

HORMONAL METHODS				
Method	Description	How it Works	Side Effects	Number of unplanned pregnancies out of 100 typical users
Injection (the Shot), Depo-Provera	Progesterone-only injection	Prevents the release of an egg and thickens the cervical mucus to prevent the passage of sperm into the uterus and may prevent implantation	Weight gain, menstrual cycle changes like irregular bleeding or spotting or amenorrhea (no period). Improves menstrual cramps and heavy bleeding. Reduces risk of uterine cancer, fibroids, anemia, PID. May decrease seizures and sickle cell anemia crises.	1 if used perfectly, 6 if not

HORMONAL METHODS						
Protection from STIs?	Prescription-only (Rx) or Over-the-counter (OTC)	Discreet	Interval of Use	Cost*	Who should use it? Anyone who:	Who should NOT use it? Anyone who:
No	Rx	Yes	Every 3 months	$35 to $75 plus office visit 4 times per year	Wants very effective temporary method that does not contain estrogen; smokers, breastfeeding women, and women over 35	Has low bone mineral density or wants to get pregnant quickly after stopping use. Anyone with current breast cancer, cardiovascular disease, lupus, migraines with aura, or other medical conditions, consult a clinician.

IMPLANTABLE CONTRACEPTION				
Method	Description	How it Works	Side Effects	Number of unplanned pregnancies out of 100 typical users
Implantable Rods (Implanon)	A plastic rod inserted under the skin of the upper arm that releases progestin over time, which alters the body's ability to get pregnant	Prevents fertilization or implantation of an egg	May cause irregular spotting, light periods, or amenorrhea (no period); lessens menstrual cramping	Less than 1
Copper Intrauterine Device, Copper T IUD, (ParaGard)	A small plastic T-shaped rod containing copper that is inserted into the uterus. The copper releases over time and alters the uterine environment.	Disables sperm, prevents fertilization, may prevent implantation	May increase menstrual flow	Less than 1

IMPLANTABLE CONTRACEPTION						
Protection from STIs?	Prescription-only (Rx) or Over-the-counter (OTC)	Discreet	Interval of Use	Cost*	Who should use it? Anyone who:	Who should NOT use it? Anyone who:
No	Rx	Maybe; rod cannot be seen but can be felt	3 to 5 years	$400 to $800, lasts 3 years	Wants a very effective long-term but temporary method or wants a method that does not contain estrogen; smokers, breastfeeding women, and women over 35	Has breast cancer, cardiovascular disease, lupus, migraine with aura, or other medical conditions, consult a clinician.
No	Rx	Yes	12 years	$500 for copper IUD, lasts 12 years		Has an abnormal uterine cavity, current or high risk for STIs, lupus, AIDS, post-transplant or other conditions, consult a clinician.

IMPLANTABLE CONTRACEPTION				
Method	Description	How it Works	Side Effects	Number of unplanned pregnancies out of 100 typical users
Hormonal IUD (Mirena, Skyla)	A small plastic T-shaped rod containing progestin that is inserted into the uterus from the vagina. The hormone releases over time and thickens the cervical mucus to prevent sperm from entering the uterus.	Thickens cervical mucus, disables sperm, may prevent ovulation and implantation	Decreases menstrual flow, may cause amenorrhea (no period)	Less than 1

IMPLANTABLE CONTRACEPTION						
Protection from STIs?	Prescription-only (Rx) or Over-the-counter (OTC)	Discreet	Interval of Use	Cost*	Who should use it? Anyone who:	Who should NOT use it? Anyone who:
No	Rx	Yes	3 to 5 years	$900 for hormonal IUD, lasts 3 years (Skyla) or 5 years (Mirena)	Wants a very effective long-term but temporary method or wants a method that does not contain estrogen; smokers, breastfeeding women, and women over 35	Has an abnormal uterine cavity, current or high risk for STIs, lupus, AIDS, post-transplant or other conditions, consult a clinician.

PERMANENT METHODS				
Method	Description	How it Works	Side Effects	Number of unplanned pregnancies out of 100 typical users
Tubal Ligation	Surgical procedure through the abdomen. The fallopian tubes are tied or clamped to permanently block the passage of egg and sperm.	Permanently prevents sperm from reaching egg	Complications of surgery - pain, bleeding; may increase risk for ectopic (tubal) pregnancy (rare)	Less than 1
Vasectomy	Surgical procedure through the scrotum to tie or clamp the vas deferens to permanently prevent sperm from entering the penis or ejaculate	Permanently prevents sperm from reaching egg	Complications of surgery - pain, bleeding	Less than 1

PERMANENT METHODS						
Protection from STIs?	Prescription-only (Rx) or Over-the-counter (OTC)	Discreet	Interval of Use	Cost*	Who should use it? Anyone who:	Who should NOT use it? Anyone who:
No	Rx	Yes	Forever	$1500 to $6000	Is sure they never want children in future. Vasectomy is much safer and less expensive than tubal ligation.	Is unsure whether they might want children in future, consult clinician.
No	Rx	Yes	Forever	$350 to $1000		

EMERGENCY CONTRACEPTION				
Method	Description	How it Works	Side Effects	Number of unplanned pregnancies out of 100 typical users
Copper IUD insertion, progestin-containing morning-after pill called ella, birth control pills	Insertion of copper IUD into the uterus from the vagina, or taking hormone-containing pills	Prevents ovulation, fertilization, or implantation	Upset stomach, lower stomach pain, vomiting, fatigue, headache, dizziness, irregular bleeding, breast tenderness	10 to 15 for pills. less than 10 for copper IUD and ella

EMERGENCY CONTRACEPTION						
Protection from STIs?	Prescription-only (Rx) or Over-the-counter (OTC)	Discreet	Interval of Use	Cost*	Who should use it? Anyone who:	Who should NOT use it? Anyone who:
No	OTC (for ages 17+), IUD requires prescription	Yes	Within 72 hours of unprotected sex	$30 to $65 for pills, $550 to $900 for IUD that lasts 12 years	Has had unprotected sex within 5 days, had a possible birth control method failure like condom breaking or forgetting to take pills, anyone who was sexually assaulted	Has had unprotected intercourse more than 5 days ago or, for the IUD, has ovulated more than 5 days ago

SOURCES:

http://www.plannedparenthood.org/

www.womenshealth.gov

www.arhp.org

www.arhp.org/uploadDocs/choosingqrg.pdf

www.webmd.com/a-to-z-guides/effectiveness-rate-of-birth-control-methods-topic-overview

Appendix II: Birth Control Method Worksheet

CHOOSING YOUR BIRTH CONTROL METHOD WORKSHEET		
Question	**Your Answer: Yes or No**	**Instructions**
Do you want to get pregnant?		If yes, circle number 1 If no, cross out number 1
Can you and your partner commit to sexual activity without having genital contact?		If yes, circle number 2 If no, cross out numbers 1 & 2
Can your partner commit to pulling out before he ejaculates? Is he able to do this every time?		If yes, circle number 3 If no, cross out number 3
Can you and your partner refrain from intercourse during the fertile time of your cycle every month? Do you have a regular cycle? Can you monitor your cycle carefully every month? If you became pregnant, could you deal with it?		If yes to all questions, circle number 4 If no to any question, cross out number 4

A more user-friendly version of this worksheet is available to download from my website: kristineshieldsauthor.com.

CHOOSING YOUR BIRTH CONTROL METHOD WORKSHEET		
Method Number	**Birth Control Methods (BCMs)**	**Notes**
1	No birth control	85 out of 100 sexually active women who use no birth control method become pregnant each year.
2	Abstinence	
3	Withdrawal	18 out of every 100 sexually active women who use withdrawal become pregnant each year.
4	Fertility awareness or natural family planning (rhythm method)	You can use a barrier method during fertile times or if your cycle becomes irregular.

CHOOSING YOUR BIRTH CONTROL METHOD WORKSHEET		
Question	**Your Answer: Yes or No**	**Instructions**
Do you want a BCM that you use only when you have intercourse?		If yes, circle numbers 5, 6, 7, & 8
Do you want protection from sexually transmitted infections?		If yes, circle number 5 or 6
Are you OK with using condoms?		If yes, circle numbers 5 & 6 If no, cross out numbers 5 & 6
Is your sex partner OK with using condoms?		If yes, circle number 6 If no, cross out number 6, but talk about number 5 (see Notes)
Are you allergic to spermicide?		If yes, cross out numbers 7 & 8
Are you OK with putting a BCM in your vagina by yourself?		If yes, circle numbers 5, 7, 8, & 11 If no, cross out numbers 5, 7, 8, & 11

CHOOSING YOUR BIRTH CONTROL METHOD WORKSHEET		
Method Number	Birth Control Methods (BCMs)	Notes
	Barrier methods	Barrier methods can be used in addition to other methods to protect against sexually transmitted infections (STIs).
		Use condoms as protection and as a BCM or use it along with your other BCM.
5	Internal (female) condom	Are you or your partner allergic to latex? Most male condoms are made of latex, but you can buy condoms made of polyurethane or animal skin. Just remember, non-latex condoms do not protect against STIs. Female condoms are not made of latex.
6	Male condom	
7	Sponge, cervical cap	Spermicide allergy is rare. Try a different brand if you are irritated by one kind.
8	Diaphragm	The diaphragm must be fitted by a clinician and requires a prescription.

CHOOSING YOUR BIRTH CONTROL METHOD WORKSHEET		
Question	**Your Answer: Yes or No**	**Instructions**
Are you OK with using hormonal methods?		If yes, circle numbers 9 through 14 If no, cross out numbers 9 through 14
Can you remember to take a pill every single day?		If yes, circle numbers 9 & 12 If no, cross out numbers 9 & 12 (see Notes)
Can you remember to change your patch once a week?		If yes, circle number 10 If no, cross out number 10
Can you remember to change your vaginal ring once a month?		If yes, circle number 11 If no, cross out number 11
Are you over 35 and a smoker?		If yes, circle numbers 12 & 13 and cross out numbers 9, 10, & 11
Are you afraid of needles?		If yes, cross out numbers 13 & 14

CHOOSING YOUR BIRTH CONTROL METHOD WORKSHEET		
Method Number	**Birth Control Methods (BCMs)**	**Notes**
	Hormonal methods	
9	Combined oral contraceptives, "the pill"	Women who should not take estrogen include smokers over 35 years old, and those who have had blood clots, certain cancers, or other diseases or cardiovascular risks. Discuss this with your health care provider.
10	Skin patch	
11	Vaginal ring (estrogen & progesterone)	
12	Progestin-only oral contraceptives, "mini-pill"	Anyone with current breast cancer, cardiovascular disease, lupus, migraine with aura, or other medical conditions should consult a health care provider before using progestin.
13	Injection (the Shot)	Fertility may not return for several months after you stop using Depo-Provera.

CHOOSING YOUR BIRTH CONTROL METHOD WORKSHEET		
Question	**Your Answer: Yes or No**	**Instructions**
Do you want to get pregnant within the next year?		If yes, cross out number 13
Can you remember to have your implant rod changed every 3 to 5 years?		If yes, circle number 14
Do you want a BCM that is highly effective, private, and reversible, that you only have to think about every 5–10 years?		If yes, circle number 15 or 16
Might you ever want to have a baby in the future?		If yes, cross out numbers 17 & 18 If no, circle numbers 17 & 18
Are you OK with having minor surgery to prevent pregnancy permanently?		If yes, circle number 17 If no, cross out number 17

CHOOSING YOUR BIRTH CONTROL METHOD WORKSHEET		
Method Number	**Birth Control Methods (BCMs)**	**Notes**
	Shot / injection (progestin-only)	Fertility may not return for several months after you stop using Depo-Provera.
	Implantable contraception	Each of these is removable by a health care provider at any time; fertility resumes immediately upon removal.
14	Implantable rod	Nexplanon contains progestin.
15	Copper IUD	ParaGard intrauterine device (IUD) contains copper, may make periods heavier.
16	Hormonal IUD	Hormonal intrauterine device (IUD) contains progestin, may make periods go away.
	Permanent methods	Surgeries to reverse these procedures are not very effective; consider them permanent.
17	Tubal ligation	Tubal ligation is performed through laparoscopic, outpatient surgery.

CHOOSING YOUR BIRTH CONTROL METHOD WORKSHEET		
Question	Your Answer: Yes or No	Instructions
Will your male partner consent to have minor surgery to prevent pregnancies?		If yes, circle number 18 If no, cross out number 18
Do you know that emergency contraceptives are available if your BCM fails, you forget to use it, or if you have intercourse against your will?		If yes, circle number 19 as a back-up method to your usual BCM If no, learn about number 19
OTHER QUESTIONS TO ASK: WHAT IS IMPORTANT TO YOU?		
Are you OK with visiting a health care provider to get a prescription for your birth control method?		If yes, all methods are available to you. If no, cross out numbers 8 through 19 and circle numbers 2 through 7
Can you afford to pay around $100 for a BCM that will last a long time?		If yes, circle numbers 14 through 18
Would you prefer to pay a small amount each time you need your BCM?		If yes, circle numbers 5 through 13

CHOOSING YOUR BIRTH CONTROL METHOD WORKSHEET		
Method Number	Birth Control Methods (BCMs)	Notes
18	Vasectomy	Vasectomy is performed in office or clinic.
19	Emergency contraception (EC)	There are no contraindications to EC. Some methods require a prescription from a health care professional. You can keep it in your cabinet in case you ever need it. Do not use as primary BCM.
OTHER QUESTIONS TO ASK: WHAT IS IMPORTANT TO YOU?		
	Requires a visit to your health care provider	Sexually active women should see a health care provider yearly for an STI exam and Pap test. (The cervical cap needs a prescription, but the sponge does not.)
	Cost	Your insurance may cover your BCM. Some clinics have free BCMs or a sliding scale fee, so you only have to pay what you can afford. More expensive methods are actually cheaper in the long run, and all BCMs are cheaper than raising a child.

CHOOSING YOUR BIRTH CONTROL METHOD WORKSHEET		
Question	Your Answer: Yes or No	Instructions
Do you want a free BCM?		If yes, circle numbers 2 through 4 (see Notes)
Do you want the most effective, reliable but temporary BCM?		If yes, circle numbers 13 through 16
Would you be OK if you had irregular bleeding or spotting between your periods?		If no, cross out numbers 9 through 14 & 16
Would you be OK if you did not have periods at all while using your BCM?		If yes, circle numbers 9, 11, 13, or 16 If no, cross out numbers 9, 11, 13, and 16
Are you at risk for uterine or ovarian cancer, ectopic pregnancy, or pelvic inflammatory disease?		If yes, circle numbers 9 through 13
Is it important that your partner does not know that you are using a BCM?		If yes, circle numbers 9, 12, 13, 15, 16, & 18

CHOOSING YOUR BIRTH CONTROL METHOD WORKSHEET		
Method Number	**Birth Control Methods (BCMs)**	**Notes**
	Cost	See previous note
	Effectiveness	
	Side effects	These methods may or may not cause you to have spotting or irregular bleeding.
		You can skip your period by taking the pill or using the ring continuously. The shot and the hormonal IUD may cause your period to stop. Not having a period is not harmful to your health.
	Contraindications	See Side Effects column in BCM Chart (Appendix I)
	Privacy	See Discreet column in BCM Chart (Appendix I)

Go back and see what numbers you have NOT crossed out. Of all the methods circled, what will work best for you? Take this chart with you to your health care provider so you can discuss your decision-making process and why you have chosen the method you did. Ask any questions you still have. Remember to protect yourself from STIs if you need to. If you're not sure you need to, you need to.

Appendix III: Birth Control Method Quiz

BCM Quiz

1. The best method of birth control for teenagers is:
   a) Birth control pills
   b) Intrauterine devices (IUDs)
   c) Condoms
   d) There is no one best method for all teenagers

2. Under the Affordable Care Act, health care insurers do not have to cover the cost of birth control methods.
   a) True
   b) False

3. After sterilization, the next most effective method of birth control is:
   a) Birth control pills
   b) Intrauterine devices (IUDs)
   c) Withdrawal
   d) The diaphragm

4. Methods of emergency contraception include:
   a) Hormonal pills
   b) Copper IUDs
   c) Neither
   d) Both

5. When is a woman least likely to get pregnant?
   a) Right before her period
   b) After breastfeeding for more than 6 months
   c) When using natural family planning
   d) When using long-acting reversible contraceptives (LARCs)

6. Which of these is not a benefit of combination birth control pills?
   a) Reduced risk of blood clots
   b) Reduced risk of certain cancers
   c) Reduced risk of ectopic pregnancy
   d) Reduced risk of pelvic inflammatory disease (PID)

7. What is the only birth control method controlled by the woman that also protects against sexually transmitted infections (STIs)?
   a) The vaginal ring
   b) The internal condom

c) The hormone shot

d) The IUD

8. Which method of birth control does not require partner agreement and cooperation?

a) The condom

b) Natural family planning

c) The hormonal implant

d) The internal condom

9. If used perfectly, which is the most effective birth control method?

a) Abstinence

b) Oral contraceptive pills

c) The hormonal patch

d) The hormone injection

10. Which is the most expensive method of family planning over a lifetime?

a) No birth control

b) Condoms

c) IUD

d) Vasectomy

Birth Control Quiz Answer Key

Give yourself one point for every correct answer.

- Scores of 9, 10: Great job!
- Scores of 7, 8: Good work!
- Scores of 4, 5, 6: Reread the sections you got wrong.
- Scores of less than 4: You might want to reread the book.

1. d. There is no best method of birth control for any age group. The right method is the one that is chosen by each individual after consideration of a number of factors. Health care providers, partners, and parents can all provide knowledge and advice, but each individual must make her own decision. But teens and young adults should consider using condoms with every episode of sexual intercourse, including oral sex, because this age group has the highest numbers of sexually transmitted infections (STIs).

2. True. The original Affordable Care Act, otherwise known as Obamacare, mandated that health insurance plans must cover birth control methods, including emergency contraceptives. But some religious organizations objected to this rule and the Supreme Court agreed that any organization that objects does not have to provide this coverage. Many insurers continue to cover the cost of BCMs, but some don't. Check your insurance plan to see if you have coverage. If you are not covered by insurance and cannot afford to pay for it, many clinics and health departments provide free or discounted services and BCMs.

3. b. The IUDs.

4. d. Both. Two kinds of hormonal pills and the copper IUD are available and effective for emergency contraception.

5. d. When using long-acting reversible contraceptive methods (LARCs). These methods include the contraceptive implants and IUDs and are the most effective methods of reversible contraception.

6. a. Reduced risk of blood clots. Using combination hormone methods can increase your risk for blood clots, and women who have had blood clots in the past should not use them.

7. b. The internal condom. Only two methods of birth control are effective against sexually transmitted infections: the male condom and the internal condom.

8. c. The hormonal implant does not require that the woman's partner know about or agree to use it.

9. a. If used PERFECTLY, abstinence is the most effective and cheapest form of birth control with the fewest side effects.

10. a. No birth control method. Over the course of your lifetime, if you do not use birth control, you will likely become pregnant. The cost of having and raising a child is more expensive than any form of birth control. The physical process of pregnancy and childbirth also carries a higher risk to your health than any form of birth control.

References

[1]U.S. Department of Disease Prevention and Health Promotion. http://www.healthypeople.gov/2020/topics-objectives/topic/family-planning. Accessed December 10, 2014.

[2]Centers for Disease Control and Prevention. Achievements in public health, 1900—1999: Family planning. MMWR Weekly. 1999 Dec 3;48(47):1073-80. Available at http://www.cdc.gov/mmwr/preview/mmwrhtml/mm4847a1.htm. Accessed December 10, 2014.

[3]Bearak J., Popinchalk A., Alkema L., and Sedgh G. Global, regional, and subregional trends in unintended pregnancy and its outcomes from 1990 to 2014: estimates from a Bayesian hierarchical model. Lancet Global Health 2018; 6:e380-89. http://dx.doi.org/10.1016/ S2214-109X(18)30029-9.

[4]Barot S. The benefits of investing in international family planning — and the price of slashing funding. Guttmacher Policy Review 2017; 20:82-85. Available at https://www.guttmacher.org/sites/default/files/article_files/gpr2008217_0.pdf.

[5]Fhi360.org. Family Planning: what and why? Handout 1. Available at https://www.fhi360.org/sites/default/files/media/documents/need-family-planning-handouts.pdf.

[6] World Health Organization. Family planning/contraception. 2018. Available at https://www.who.int/news-room/fact-sheets/detail/family-planning-contraception.

[7] Curtis K.M., Jatlaoui T.C., Tepper N.K., et al. U.S. selected recommendations for contraceptive use, 2016. MMWR Recomm Rep 2016; 65(No. RR-4):1-66. DOI: http://dx.doi.org/10.15585/mmwr.rr6504a1.

[8] Planned Parenthood. http://www.plannedparenthood.org/about-us/newsroom/press-releases/ten-little-known-facts-about-condoms-planned-parenthood#shash.IL-nORymw.dpuf. Accessed December 10, 2014.

[9] Association of Reproductive Health Professionals. https://www.arhp.org/Publications-and-Resources/Quick-Reference-Guide-for-Clinicians/choosing/Vaginal-Ring. Accessed December 10, 2014.

[10] Guttmacher Institute. 2018. Contraceptive Use in the United States. https://www.guttmacher.org/fact-sheet/contraceptive-use-united-states.

[11] U.S. Department of Health and Human Services. Emergency contraception. Accessed March 19, 2020 at https://www.hhs.gov/opa/pregnancy-prevention/birth-control-methods/emergency-contraception/index.html.

[12] Spotnitz M.E., Natarajan K., Ryan P. & Westhoff C.L. Relative risk of cervical neoplasms among copper and levonorgestrel-releasing intrauterine system users. Obstetrics & Gynecology 2020; 135(2):310-327. doi: 10.1097/AOG.0000000000003656.

[13]Adolescents and long-acting reversible contraception: implants and intrauterine devices. Committee Opinion No. 539. American College of Obstetricians and Gynecologists. Obstet Gynecol 2012; 120:983—8. Available at http://www.acog.org/Resources-And-Publications/Committee-Opinions/Committee-on-Adolescent-Health-Care/Adolescents-and-Long-Acting-Reversible-Contraception. Accessed December 10, 2014.

[14] Em M. Male birth control: current options and new breakthroughs. The Checkup, August 6, 2018. Available at https://www.singlecare.com/blog/male-birth-control-options/. Accessed 27July2020.

[15]Planned Parenthood. http://www.plannedparenthood.org/health-info/morning-after-pill-emergency-contraception#sthash.avzfK1nA.dpuf. Accessed December 10, 2014.

[16]U.S. Department of Health and Human Services. Emergency contraception. Accessed March 19, 2020 at https://www.hhs.gov/opa/pregnancy-prevention/birth-control-methods/emergency-contraception/index.html.

[17]U.S. Department of Agriculture. http://www.usda.gov/wps/portal/usda/usdahome?contentidonly=true&contentid=2014/08/0179.xml. Accessed December 10, 2014.

[18]Cleland, Kelly; Peipert, Jeffrey F.; Westhoff, Carolyn; Spear, Scott; Trussell, James (2011). "Family Planning as a Cost-Saving Preventive Health Service." New England Journal of Medicine; 364(18):e37.

Author's Note

I would like to acknowledge the following people and organizations for their support of me through my career in women's health.

Planned Parenthood Federation of America — who created and operated one of the first certificate programs for women's health nurse practitioners. In doing so, they provided well-educated, committed, and passionate health care providers who assisted women with their reproductive health care needs, and who often became their patients' primary care providers. PPFA's dedication to inclusion, diversity, empowerment, and reproductive justice shaped much more than my career. Miriam Manisoff and Sandy Worthington were tireless advocates for nurse practitioner education and women's health.

Planned Parenthood of Southeastern Pennsylvania — who sponsored me in the NP program, hired me in my first NP position, and introduced me to the world of reproductive health and reproductive rights. I've been dedicated to the mission ever since. To all of my fellow women's health nurse practitioners, educators and administrators who taught me, led me, and supported me in my practice and in my life. Special thanks to Mary Banecker, Barbara Kubiak, and Barbara Rinto.

To the folks who helped me write this book, including Esther Desher CRNP for early review, Diana Sinovic for editing, Jill Angel for proofreading, the Noun Project and

Romy Spekreijse for the icons, Sarah Beaudin for the design, Chloe Shields, Katie and Grace Horigan for beta readings, and the woman who inspired the book, Elizabeth Hanes, nurse writer par excellence.

Finally, to my kids: Nick, Chloe, and John, to my partner Walter, and to my mom, who died last year. Thank you for supporting me, grounding me, and surrounding me with love, no matter what.

Free Gift

NOTE: Don't forget to head over to my website at www.kristineshieldsauthor.com to request a FREE downloadable BCM worksheet to fill out yourself or to share.

Author Biography

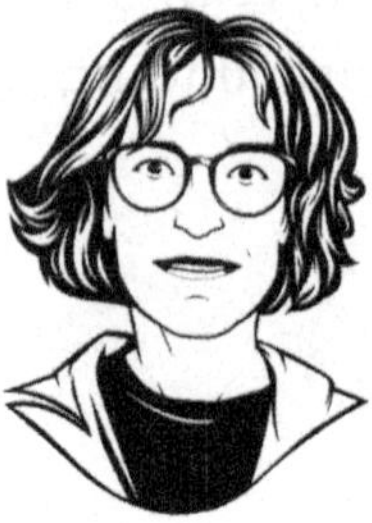

Kristine Shields MSN, DrPH, is a Women's Health Nurse Practitioner with a doctoral degree in Public Health. Women's health and empowerment issues motivated her career as a women's health clinician and public health professional.

Dr. Shields worked at Planned Parenthood and other women's clinics in the Philadelphia area, including a drug treatment program for women and an HMO for jail and prison inmates.

She is a Perspectives Editor for the BMJ journal *Sexually Transmitted Infections* and has published papers in *Obstetrics & Gynecology*, *Pediatrics*, *Birth Defects Research* and other journals.

Having worked in drug safety and ethics within a pharmaceutical company for many years, in 2019 she published "Pregnancy and the Pharmaceutical Industry: The Movement Towards Evidence-Based Pharmacotherapy for Pregnant Women."

In wishing to improve access to reproductive health care, Dr. Shields is currently publishing a series of guidebooks about women's health issues. The next in this series is *The*

Vulva Owner's Manual on Medical Abortion and Emergency Contraception. Her next full book, tentatively titled *My Life in STIs: Destigmatizing the Hidden Epidemic*, is targeted for publication in 2021.

Dr. Shields lives and writes in Bucks County, PA, but is frequently sighted in Charleston, SC. She can be reached at Kristine@kristineshieldsauthor.com, and you can visit her website or sign up to receive her monthly newsletter, Paddendum, at www.kristineshieldsauthor.com.

Please share your questions, comments, and updates with Dr. Shields on her website at www.kristineshieldsauthor.com or follow her on:

- **LinkedIn:** www.linkedin.com/in/kristineshieldsdrph
- **Twitter:** www.twitter@KShieldsauthor
- **Medium:** https://medium.com/@kristineshieldsauthor
- **Amazon:** http://bit.ly/KESAuthor

Made in the USA
Monee, IL
04 November 2026

67387873R00085